Publisher's Note
The information in this book is not intended to be taken as a replacement for medical advice. Any person with a condition requiring medical attention should consult a qualified medical practitioner or suitable therapist. The directions for treatment of particular diseases are given for the guidance of medical practitioners only, and should not be prescribed by those who do not have a medical training

Sergio Maria Francardo

Anthroposophic Medicine for all the Family
Recognizing and treating
common disorders

RUDOLF STEINER PRESS

Rudolf Steiner Press
Hillside House, The Square
Forest Row, RH18 5ES

www.rudolfsteinerpress.com

First published in English translation by Edilibri srl, 2013
This edition published by Rudolf Steiner Press, 2017

© Rudolf Steiner Press, 2017

The editor thanks Dr. Frank Mulder
for his valuable help and support

Originally published under the title *Medicina antroposofica familiare. Riconoscere e curare le malattie più comuni* by Edilibri srl, Milano, 2004

Translated from Italian by Rachel Stenner / LCC
© Edilibri srl, 2013

This book is copyright under the Berne Convention. All rights reserved. Apart from any fair dealing for the purpose of private study, research, criticism or review, no part of this publication may be reproduced, stored in a retrieval system, or transmitted in any form or by any means, electronic, electrical, chemical, mechanical, optical, photocopying, recording or otherwise, without the prior written permission of the copyright owner. Inquiries should be addressed to the Publishers

The right of Sergio Maria Francardo to be identified as the author of this work has been asserted in accordance with sections 77 and 78 of the Copyright, Designs and Patents Act, 1988

A CIP catalogue record for this book is available from the British Library

Print book ISBN: 978 1 85584 534 3
Ebook ISBN: 978 1 85584 494 0

Cover by Morgan Creative
Typeset by Edilibri srl, Milan
Printed and bound by 4Edge Ltd., Essex

Contents

7 Preface
by Dr. Giancarlo Buccheri

PART ONE
General notions
13 Anthroposophic medicine
21 The four constituent parts of the human being
24 The functional threefoldness of humans
26 Health and illness
34 Fever and the warmth body
39 The importance of nutrition to health in childhood

PART TWO
Illnesses and remedies
52 How to deal with a fever
57 Colds and cold-related illnesses
62 Influenza
68 Sore throat
75 Subglottic laryngitis or false croup
77 Sinusitis
84 The cough: an unwelcome defence mechanism
96 The prevention and treatment of allergies
107 Hay fever
114 Asthma
125 Conjunctivitis: the weeping eye
129 Earache
133 Dental disorders
138 Headache: when the head hurts
143 Bloating and flatulence: wind imprisoned by the metabolism
147 Abdominal pain

159	Diarrhoea
165	Traveller's diarrhoea and summer food poisoning
169	Constipation: holding nature within us
175	Haemorrhoids and anal fissures
180	Varicose veins and phlebitis
183	A change of air
186	Enuresis: the wet bed
189	Cystitis and urethritis
200	Menstrual pain (dysmenorrhoea)
203	Impetigo
205	Shingles: *Herpes zoster*
208	Cold sores: *Herpes simplex*
213	Warts: an unpleasant manifestation
217	Acne and boils
221	Eczema and dermatitis
230	Bites and stings
233	Sunburn
235	Burns and scalds
237	Trauma and surgery
245	Rheumatism and joint pain: an obstacle to movement
251	Muscle cramps
253	Torticollis: a praise of slowness
257	Low back pain: lumbago
263	Childhood illnesses
272	Tiredness: giving way to the forces of weight
280	Anaemia: the strength of Mars to stay on the Earth
288	Sleep disorders and anxiety
302	Hypertension: the silent killer

APPENDIX

317	The household medicine store
323	Information on anthroposophic medicine
325	Bibliography
329	Subject index

Preface
by Dr. Giancarlo Buccheri [1]

It is with great pleasure that I present this manual of anthroposophic medicine for family use, written by my dear colleague Sergio Maria Francardo.
Almost one hundred years have passed since anthroposophic medicine was inaugurated in central Europe when in 1920, in Dornach, Rudolf Steiner held a first cycle of medical lectures. By 1921 Dr. Ita Wegman was able to open a small clinic near Basel, with the aim of verifying the validity of Steiner's spiritual insights in a clinical setting.
Since then anthroposophic medicine has spread throughout the world, being taken up by ever larger groups of patients, doctors and therapists who find in its spiritual foundations a valid, modern response to the deeper questions underlying illness and healing. Ita Wegman, of Dutch origin, was particularly keen that anthroposophic medicine would take root in the English speaking world. She travelled frequently to Great Britain to encourage English colleagues to open clinics, treatment centres and homes for children with special needs. In addition, through her international friendships, she sought to promote anthroposophic medicine in North America.
Sergio Maria Francardo shows how the anthroposophic medical impulse can unfold in a country with historical, cultural and social backgrounds very different from those in which anthroposophic

---

[1] Former President of the International Federation of Anthroposophic Medical Associations.

medicine began, showing that anthroposophy is not a doctrine, but a way of learning. Therefore, its character changes depending on the individual and the cultural setting in which it is received. Just as a diamond reflects the light from all its facets, so anthroposophy, if lived with consistency and dedication, can mirror the results of an individual's inner journey. However, unlike the diamond, anthroposophy is enriched and grows precisely by virtue of the light we bring to it.

Without claiming to be exhaustive, the author wishes to make the fruits of his personal experience, accumulated over several decades of practice in a large Italian city (Milan), available not only to his colleagues, but to all who are interested. He has, therefore, chosen to use plain and transparent language such as every doctor strives to use with his patients, rather than scholarly formulations, but without loss of scientific precision.

Through the individual chapters we are led by the author not so much in the discovery of particular remedies, but rather the deeper aspects of a given illness. Beyond the immediate help to relieve suffering, doctors are often asked about the possible meaning of such suffering in the span of an individual's biography or in a social context.

Exploring these questions involves patient and doctor in a close therapeutic relationship. This stands at the heart of anthroposophic medicine as one of the highest duties of a doctor.

Some charming autobiographical references are scattered through the single chapters, showing that the author still loves his profession, which has enabled him to provide concrete help to many suffering people and has enhanced his own moral development.

Besides precise descriptions of single treatments suited to a home setting, we can draw from the pearls of wisdom contained in this

Preface

manual a wider view of medicine: one that should not be experienced only as an abstract set of scientific or statistical data, but that embraces a human and personal story in which both patient and doctor are conscious participants.

Our gratitude goes to Sergio Maria Francardo, and we hope that his commitment as an anthroposophic doctor brings him many more valuable experiences, which he will no doubt want to share with us in future.

(G.B.)

To my wife, Evelina

PART ONE

General notions

Introductory note
Anthroposophic medicine originated around the 1920s, building on the requests of medical disciples of Rudolf Steiner (1861-1925), the founder of anthroposophy, a school of thought and spiritual research also called *spiritual science*. It was precisely the scientific approach to research that gave rise to the numerous practical applications of anthroposophy that spread throughout the world, such as biodynamic agriculture, the anthroposophic Waldorf educational system, living organic architecture and new forms of art, including eurythmy as the art of visible speech. Ita Wegman, a doctor who was very close to Steiner and who wanted to give impetus to the movement of anthroposophic medicine, founded, with Steiner's support, the first clinic of anthroposophic medicine in Arlesheim (Basel, Switzerland). The clinic, now named the "Ita Wegman Klinik", still exists. It does, therefore, seem wholly justified to state that anthroposophic medicine was born at the patient's bedside: in welcoming their first patients, the anthroposophic doctors experienced the enormous potential that this medical system offers for empathic support of the person who is suffering. There are currently numerous anthroposophic clinics and large hospitals particularly in Switzerland, Germany, the Netherlands, Sweden and England. Contemporaneously there was a surge in interest in anthroposophic medicines, aimed at producing new drugs for the clinic and its patients; this interest led to the creation of a huge range of remedies produced by major pharmaceutical companies such as the Weleda and the Wala, which have production plants in the numerous countries in the world in which anthroposophic medicine is widespread. Information on anthroposophic medicine and medicinal products can be found on the website of the International Federation of Anthroposophic Medical Associations (*www.ivaa.info*).

Anthroposophic medicine

The distinction between mainstream and non-conventional medicine is still the subject of lively debate and, indeed, disagreement. Here we want to concentrate on what characterizes the philosophy of anthroposophic medicine which, in a scientific context, is not limited to acquiring knowledge, but is extended to give particular attention to a correct inner attitude.

Compared to mainstream medicine which, in a manner considered scientific, starts from a certain image or idea of matter to arrive at the human being, anthroposophic medicine, in a different but equally scientific way, starts from the human being to approach nature, life and matter. The driving force of this different approach is to promote the human aspect of medicine, integrating and remedying the "coldest" aspects of the technology used in this field. Anthroposophic medicine, which was founded in a hospital, neither opposes nor negates classical physiology, but tries to extend it following a precise method of research, comparable to that of classical science.

In concrete terms, anthroposophic medicine asks the doctor for efforts of self-education, to try to develop perceptive faculties able to broaden his consciousness and make it more sensitive to areas of research that are no less real than the phenomena studied in medical school. The task proposed is to refine the perceptive organs, just as the cardiologist refines his hearing, the surgeon his sense of touch and the radiologist his sight.

The anthroposophic doctor must, therefore, develop a specific perception of the vital processes within the body, of the psychological (soul) realities related to bodily existence and, finally, of those individual elements which combine with the physical, vital and soul components forming a whole. For those who want to embrace it, the anthroposophic approach *exacts* a precise research methodology, has its own study criteria and uses its own terminology. Like any other field of science, anthroposophic spiritual science has a specific discipline, without which reasonable results cannot be reached, just as no-one can expect that a person without mathematical training would be able to deal with quantum physics.

I would like to emphasize that this methodology is based on the results that Rudolf Steiner himself obtained by applying his method of spiritual-scientific research. Steiner never practiced medicine directly, but the fruits of his research were bestowed on doctors who started to use them under his spiritual guidance.

This spiritual-scientific methodology broadened the boundaries of natural sciences thanks to precise knowledge of the spiritual world and gave rise to numerous concrete achievements. I shall mention only one here: biodynamic agriculture. This is an anthroposophic husbandry of the land that is obtaining exceptional results in the most difficult situations. For example, in Australia more than two million hectares of land desertified by industrial livestock management and intensive agriculture have been brought back to life. In the light of these results, the Australian government has included an expert in biodynamics among its representatives at the major world conferences on the health of the Earth, such as the one held in Rio de Janeiro in 1992 and the one in South Africa in 2002.

Rudolf Steiner developed a system of self-education that offers the basis for approaching the knowledge that we described earlier: it is the lodestone for all doctors wanting to pursue anthroposophic medicine. This form of medicine tries to give importance not only to those tangible, objectifiable, measurable, weighable and numerically expressible findings in a sick patient or an impaired organ with its altered values, but also to those elements that express the soul, character and biographical aspects of each individual, including the social and cultural environment in order to combine all these factors when making a therapeutic choice.

Uniting these areas of existence and realities with diagnostic considerations and related observations, we are faced with unique, *individual constellations* of conditions.

A pre-determined therapeutic regimen is, therefore, rarely of help[2]. For example, all patients who develop pneumonia have some typical symptoms such as fever, cough, production of phlegm (sputum), pain, malaise, myalgia, altered blood-chemistry values with raised levels of inflammation markers in the blood (such as the erythrocyte sedimentation rate or ESR), and characteristic signs on a chest X-ray. However, every patient experiences the disease in his own way; that is, the disease has a different meaning for each person. Each one is torn in some way from the fabric of his life, professional activity or family. One patient may suffer only from this disease, whereas another may experience it as a secondary event or as a consequence of a tumour or a surgical operation. One patient may have considerable reserves of strength, whereas another may have already been debilitated before becoming ill. One patient may be young, with small children, and wants to get well quickly; another who is old, alone and self-sufficient until becoming sick, would rather die than have to go to a hospice after his illness and does not, therefore, know whether he really wants to get better. *Every patient with pneumonia lacks something specific to feel healthy again, to regain a harmonious relationship with his surroundings.*

Although drugs are the necessary basis for every medical prescription, the choice depends on the specific disease, its severity, stage, whether it is acute or chronic, the age of the patient, the patient's reserves of strength, his constitution, and collaboration in the healing process. Furthermore, prescriptions are subject to the conception that a doctor has of a disease. For instance, if the doctor considers that bacteria are the sole cause of the pneumonia, he will prescribe an antibiotic as a targeted treatment. An anthroposophic doctor may also have to prescribe antibiotics, for example when treating a very debilitated, elderly or frightened

---

[2] Every dogmatism is rejected by anthroposophic medicine and so while the ideal is a search for personalised treatment, on the other hand one of the strengths of the anthroposophic range of remedies is that it includes drugs for typical diseases which are aimed at strengthening an organ or reinforcing a function, which will often be referred to in this book.

patient. I would, however, like to point out that every year between 40,000 and 70,000 people die of pneumonia in the USA, with this disease ranking sixth among the leading causes of death and being the most common fatal infection acquired in hospital. *To say that antibiotics have eliminated death from pneumonia seems to be rather triumphalistic.*

Alternatively, the doctor can consider the spread of bacteria in the airways and lungs as the consequence of an alteration in the balance of forces within the sick body, where fluids filter from the blood through the walls of the alveoli, invading the space normally occupied by air and creating a fertile environment for bacterial proliferation. In this case, the doctor will try to restore the balance of forces by eliminating the primary alteration and stimulating the patient's self-healing powers.

For example, to counteract the loss of warmth from the chest, we can apply external remedies that release warmth, such as *poultices*, or we can prescribe anti-inflammatory treatments for internal use, such as *phosphorus*; furthermore, the patient can be given *potentised iron* to stimulate the respiratory process, *antimony* to restore order to the proteins that have burst out of cells into the interstitial fluids, or other drugs in homeopathic doses, such as *aconite* and *bryony*, to rebalance the organic liquids (we speak of the "fluid body"). Anthroposophic medicine has its specific pharmacopoeia based on the use of minerals, metals and plants appropriately processed for pharmaceutical use.

Rudolf Steiner gave a new system to the identification of medicines. He described the evolutionary relationships between mankind and nature's kingdoms in an entirely novel way, shedding some light on these connections which do, of course, require long study and refinement to be understood. Minerals, plants and animals can be studied and understood in the same way that man is studied and understood. We have to find the "key" to give each patient that specific something that he lacks, that flower which does not bloom or grows poorly in "his garden", or that mineral which will re-invigorate "his ground". This means applying a qualitative form of observation, examining the qualities of living

Anthroposophic medicine

and sentient beings: their characteristics, properties and forms of expression in the physical, chemical, biological, spatial and temporal environment. Collectively these phenomena manifest the active powers related to the essential nature of a plant, a mineral or a metal. A medicine identified in this way from nature's kingdoms can then be used appropriately for treatment.

Whether you want to supply warmth or reduce it, relieve a cramp, or stimulate or slow down the metabolism, nature always has a valuable remedy: the problem is simply to find it.

The anthroposophic doctor obviously also prescribes conventional drugs, for example a hormone replacement therapy such as insulin in the case of diabetes. In general, however, preference is given to medicines derived from nature, since their therapeutic relationship with man is linked to their common origin. These remedies are activated through various different pharmaceutical processes, some very complex, which are typical of anthroposophic medicine.

The substances are used in precisely targeted ways to act on one or other of the functional systems differentiated in anthroposophic medicine; the choice of medicinal plants does not depend only on the active ingredients that they contain, but also on their conditions of growth and cultivation as well as on the methods used in their pharmaceutical processing.

For example, if I want to act on the *nerve-sense system*, which is at the very core of man's inner life and concerns the sphere of *thinking*, I would use a remedy *applied externally*, such as a compress, and if I use a plant I would choose its *roots*. Thought, of course, could be trained and *strengthened by exercising it* sufficiently.

If I want to act on the *metabolic-limb system* – digestion and the locomotor apparatus – which are the basis of *volition*, I would use a remedy *taken into the body*, such as tablets or drops, and if I use a plant I would choose its *flowers* or *fruit*. Dealing with the metabolism, if I want to educate the system, I would use strategies involving the *diet* and a healthy approach to *movement*.

Finally, to act on the *rhythmic system* – mainly the respiratory and cardiovascular systems – which underlie *feelings*, I would make use of a treatment *injected* subcutaneously or intravenously, choosing the *leaves* or *stem* of a plant; I would prescribe *art* and *artistic therapies* to cure the *emotional state*, to restore the right rhythm to the tumult of emotions. Art experienced concretely by the soul has a completely different effect from art simply thought about or reproduced from a book or video, which really only affects thinking.

It would be too restrictive to consider anthroposophic medicine only as a therapeutic approach that uses natural remedies. Rather, it is a discipline that strives to understand experiences in a broader framework, integrating them into a scientific representation of the relationship between man and nature, aspiring to the ideal of identifying the specific remedy for each condition. This remedy could be a natural cure, a conventional treatment, a conversation, one of the marvellous *anthroposophic artistic therapies* or *eurythmy*, the art of movement that can activate the forces underlying the intrinsic laws of language and musical sounds, important for disorders of the locomotor apparatus, such as scoliosis, sight, hearing and language and so wonderful in the treatment of disabled children. What amazes visitors to the Lukas Klinik, an anthroposophic clinic for the treatment of cancer near Basel in Switzerland, is seeing assiduously engaged people moving from one occupation to another, sitting next to them in the clinic's restaurant and then discovering that they are patients, severely ill with cancer. In anthroposophic medicine activities such as art therapy or going to the theatre are considered equally important as an injection or a pill.

I still remember my feeling of joy and wonder when, as a young and inexperienced doctor, I saw a seriously ill patient with cancer at the Lukas Klinik coming out of a session of watercolour painting with flushed cheeks and enthusiastically showing me his pictures: a quantum leap from the lung cancer ward that I frequented in Milan, where I saw only pale faces in a black and white world. I must be clear that any doctor who, working in the setting of traditional medicine, cares for a patient with devotion and uses his knowledge to alleviate suffering, deserves the greatest respect. The criticism that could be raised is on a philosophical level, that materialistic thinking, supported by more than a century of positivism, cannot see anything beyond molecules. And yet, already a century ago, modern physics had surpassed a world restricted to molecules and atoms: in fact, there are an infinite number of realities and we humans only perceive a minuscule part of them. Just consider radiation or sounds, of which we perceive only an infinitesimal fraction. We must emerge from the barrenness of the laboratory and behold the marvellous, infinite and glittering colours of a diamond held up to the light: in the dark or from a molecular point of view it is only a fossil, a lump of carbon!

A knowledge-based attitude refuses to appreciate that a smile can be a better treatment than a psychoactive drug. The innocent stare of a child can harmonise our soul and, like the baton of a conductor, reaching the engine room of biochemistry, guide the whole orchestra of neurotransmitters that govern our nervous system: that emotion observed, despite the absence of physical molecules, operates profoundly. The gentle effects of anthroposophic remedies are thwarted and lost if the doctor lacks devotion to humanity.

Let me give you a practical example: modern medicine, to which I belong, boasts of having reduced deaths due to hypertension. Take a 40- or 50-year old man, who often has a harmful lifestyle and simply tell him to eat less salt and fried food, renouncing attempts to take really incisive measures, even if arduous, such as a completely reformulated diet or perhaps joining dancing classes. The man is prescribed an antihypertensive drug which he will have to take for his whole life. In the future, as he gets older, he will very probably have to take other antihypertensive treatments, but in the meantime he continues with his bad habits. One day, when he has a small stroke he will be reprimanded for having forgotten to take his life-saving pill, while his existence becomes colourless and he sees himself turning grey. Then he will become a faithful husband, perhaps because his blood pressure tablets have made him impotent, and before long he will be a client for new drugs proposed to restore his sex life. He will be unable to be stirred by a concert, because this would involve an emotion that would increase his heart rate, which his beta-blocker drug does not allow. He will gradually become a burden on the conscience of his children who, without knowing it, are following his same path. Swallowing pill after pill, he will end up waiting for his postponed death in a hospice, where he has been consigned by his inability to perceive his own emotions and a society that does not have time for people who suffer. Many of you perhaps already know Tolstoy's story of a child who sees his parents give his elderly, weak grandfather food in a wooden bowl, no longer considering him worthy of pottery. Shortly afterwards, they see their child carving some wood. When they ask him, "What are you doing?", he replies, "I am preparing a bowl for when you are old!"

If life loses its quality, saving it saves absolutely nothing, it is simply a hoax: a prophylactic against vascular death. I have seen men literally bloom after having had the courage to abandon soul-constricting treatment.

Recovering a life worth living: this is real quality of life!

The four constituent parts of the human being

A person's quality of life can be preserved by observing and treating the individual as a whole, taking into account that the human being consists of a physical body, an ether body, an astral body and "I". This differentiation of the human being made by anthroposophy enables us to understand that each part of the human being can be affected by a disease. It is essential to consider that the manifold nature of a disease can help us establish sensible rules and therapeutic strategies. Let's look briefly now at the four constituent parts of the human being.

The physical body
The *physical body* is the only visible part of man and is composed of the *solid* substances of the external world. Its shape and functional connections are inexplicable in themselves, because an upright posture, feeling, looking, thinking, wanting, etc. are not consequences of physicality but are expressions of a soul-spirit element in continuous evolution in the body. The physical body is kept alive by vital forces; if it is abandoned by these forces, it succumbs to the laws of the mineral world, as happens to corpses. Merely by understanding this obvious concept, one can already accept the existence of life forces. Spiritual science invites us to understand this system of intangible forces, invisible to the physical eye, which is structured and shaped as a life body.

The ether body or life body
Man has an *ether body*, just as plants do. This ether body underlies the phenomena of growth and reproduction, stimulates and orientates metabolism, overcomes the weight of the solid matter of the physical body, models it as a sculptor does with clay, creating a shape according to an archetypical personal structure, and introduces it into a higher order: that of the vital forces. The moulding vital forces work in *liquids*. In fact, there is no life without water. There are differences in the vital processes between

plants, animals and humans. In fact, plants can form organic substances from inorganic ones, while animals and humans require a supply of organic substances from the exterior.

The astral body or soul body
The *astral body* is the "sentient body", the carrier of pain and pleasure, of passions and emotions. In brief, this means that it has a soul life. Consciousness and a soul life mark the transition from plant to animal. Animals and humans owe their soul life in part to their capacity for autonomous movement, of being, in fact, "animated". The higher order principle of this organization is the sphere of sensation or feeling, which includes sympathy, antipathy, impulses and instincts, but also consciousness. Consciousness enables human beings both to collect information provided by the senses and to capture the spiritual element of thought, that is to say, to recognize the laws of nature and the cosmos.

As the ether body gives shape, by acting on fluids in rhythmic movement, so the astral body is united with the body by means of the *gaseous* or aeriform component: it modulates its hold on bodily existence through the dual movements of respiration.

The organization of "I"
The fourth component making up a human being is the "I", the faculty of self-awareness, which is the stage of evolution reached only by humans. A being who can say "I" to himself has within him his own personal world perceivable in his way of thinking, acting and feeling emotions. A spiritual element, to which he can learn to feel responsible and committed, develops within him. It is that voice of conscience that nowadays we so skilfully silence with the thundering sound and illusory glitter of modern life. Even in the doctor's waiting room, where we could finally be in peace with ourselves for a bit, we are greeted by idiotic tunes and obtuse magazines encouraging us to be part of the unreal private life of VIPs.

The "I" creates a real "organization of I" in the body; permeating deeply into an area that is well beyond wakeful consciousness,

The four constituent parts of the human being

it shapes individual functional and structural body systems on a human scale. No human body is identical to another; this personal imprint even penetrates physical matter. This has been demonstrated by molecular biology, which has shown us that each individual, starting from his own genes, creates a personal set of proteins and we can say that there are as many different proteins in the world as there are human beings!

Warmth is the element that, through its organic vehicle (blood), opens the world of matter to the "I". It is not for nothing that Mephistopheles asks Faust to sign in blood. It expresses the eternal individuality (entelechy) of the human being.

Steiner's anthropology urges us to look at man taking into account his complexity and his intimate needs. This broadened image of man is a keystone of anthroposophic philosophy, whose teaching, based on this image, is intended to promote healthy and serene development of the child, so that he can become a free man. I am profoundly struck, in that courageous and strenuous utopia of a Waldorf school, by the fact that a carpentry teacher may make such profound considerations about a child that sometimes not even the anthroposophic doctor or the class teacher could have understood about the child's personality. Castes are overcome: the "High priest" of the classroom and the medical "General" must bow to the manual worker, to the "untouchable", to the bearer of a knowledge that they do not have.

Such a man, well rooted in the four constituent parts with his manual creativity that cannot be replaced by any machine, gives me hope for our future.

Let's recapitulate schematically the four-fold nature of man in relation to the states of matter and the kingdoms of nature.

Constituent of man	*State of matter*	*Nature's kingdom*
PHYSICAL BODY	Solid	Mineral
ETHER BODY	Liquid	Vegetable
ASTRAL BODY	Gaseous	Animal
"I"	Warmth	Human

The functional threefoldness of humans

The understanding that man is a quadripartite being, explained in the preceding chapter, is completed and deepened by knowledge of the three principles acting in each of the four constituent parts of humans and in the universe:
– the principle of shape or of solidification: the *nerve-sense system*;
– the principle of entering into solution or dissolution: the *metabolic-limb system*;
– the principle of mediation or balance: the *rhythmic system*.

The nerve-sense system
Within the physical body, the nerve-sense system can be distinguished as the pole of calm. It supports the formation of thoughts as the result of the encounter between our sensory perceptions and our thinking activity. Through sensory perception we can compare and relate ourselves to the external world, developing our own thoughts. We speak of a formative process which has its physiological basis in the brain, neurosensory system and the sensory organs. The vitality of these organs regresses very early and they lose the capacity to reproduce and grow: they hardly regenerate any more.
We live each day spending our "share of neurones" in processes of wakeful consciousness. Here is the basis of the physical activity of thinking. Man's consciousness is manifested in a formative process which is supported at the expense of life in the opposite pole, the metabolic-limb system.

The metabolic-limb system
In this pole of movement, processes of transformation and regeneration predominate. External substances are converted into the body's own substances. Here the confrontation and connection with matter is determined. These processes occur completely below the threshold of consciousness and constitute the phys-

ical support for the will, the faculty to act that can be expressed through the metabolism and the organs of movement.

The rhythmic system
The processes described above, which are opposites, are kept in equilibrium by the mediation of rhythmic processes. This mediation enables the irreconcilable polar processes of calm (shape) and motion (dissolution) to act regularly in the body. The physiological basis of the rhythmic system is provided by the cardiovascular apparatus and the lungs, but wherever a rhythmic process, such as the activity of the digestive tract, occurs, the rhythmic system is brought into play. This system continuously balances the two poles. It constitutes the basis for interpreting the life of feelings, the emotions.

Let's summarise the relations between the three-fold organization of the human being, his soul activity, alchemical processes, plants and man's spirit:

	Physical man	*Soul activity*	*Alchemical process*	*Plant*	*Spiritual man*
Nerve-sense system	HEAD	THINKING	SALT	ROOT	PAST
Rhythmic system	CHEST	FEELING	MERCURY	LEAF	PRESENT
Metabolic-limb system	ABDOMEN/ LIMBS	VOLITION	SULPHUR	FLOWER	FUTURE

These three principles operate in all the constituent parts of the human being. From this point of view, illness is a disturbance in the balance between these three principles.
On the psychological level, which the anthroposophic doctor prefers to call soul, they implement the three faculties of thinking, feeling and volition, whereas at the level of the "I", or the spirit, they express the faculties of memory, self-awareness and planning existence (past, present and future).

Health and illness

In human beings two forces are at work in both health and illness: nature, i.e., the physical body that is part of the sensible world (the world that can be perceived by our senses), and the spirit, man's soul-spiritual being that belongs to the supersensible world (the world beyond the perception of our sensory organs). Two worlds face each other: the natural world – bearer of the mineral-forming wisdom and the sacrificial force[3] necessary for life on Earth, which is manifested in the instinct and physico-chemical laws that regulate the body – and the spirit world, of moral and spiritual values, represented by the "I" of man, which is expressed in the uniqueness of every human being.

There was a very acute awareness of this duality in illness in ancient times, when disease was not so much a question of natural science as a religious problem. In fact, we know that medicine was founded in temples. The ancient healers believed that illness was a consequence of sin. It is sufficient to read the book of *Genesis*, or watch some traditional sacred plays to understand that the original sin, the devil's temptation, was considered the origin of disease.

Modern science has reversed the terms of the problem, reaching, through the genetic determinism of molecular biology, the conclusion that sin comes from disease, from an exchange of amino acids in the double chain of the DNA that conveys information from the centre of a cell. This scientific conception claims that man is a morally neutral being and the fact that he behaves in one way or another derives from characteristics of his bodily make

---

[3] A fundamental teaching of anthroposophy is the concept that evolution is based on love and sacrifice. Over the ages some spiritual beings have been sacrificed in order that others could evolve; this sacrifice creates a deep bond between humans and nature's other beings. The future task of mankind is to promote, through its own sacrifice, the evolution of beings that allowed humans to reach the top: we must be grateful to the spiritual beings "represented" by minerals, plants and animals.

up. It is naively thought that Lombroso's external materialism[4] has been abandoned, but believing – as Lombroso did – that criminal behaviours could be recognized from a certain shape of skull is not very different, from a perspective of freedom, from identifying them through genetic traits.

The two conceptions, religious and scientistic[5], are both one-sided, whereas we must understand that two worlds are involved in sickness and health: the natural world, represented by man's body, and the spiritual world, represented by the soul-spirit individuality of the person.

A purely physical conception is not, therefore, able to understand sickness, because one of the terms of the equation, that is, the inner life, is seen only as an expression and consequence of physical processes that take place in the human being, in particular those occurring in the brain. The other term of the equation, the moral and spiritual world, completely loses its reality, becoming something nebulous and virtual, a type of smoke arising from metabolic processes of the brain.

---

[4] Cesare Lombroso (Verona 1835 - Turin 1909) an Italian psychiatrist and anthropologist. Founder of criminal anthropology, he believed he could identify *somatic traits* that distinguished criminals. This mechanistic research approach was superseded and quickly considered grotesque. There was a significant meeting between Lombroso and Tolstoy, in which there was a complete lack of comprehension between the great author, overflowing with love for humanity, and the scientist, concentrating on searching for the traits of genius in Tolstoy's face.

[5] We use the term 'scientific' to indicate the attitude of thought of those who subordinate every possible human condition or activity to an empirical, measurable factor. Although this attitude has led to great advances in modern medicine, it carries the serious risk of reducing man to a very complicated machine. Many times we doctors are led to decide that, in a particular patient, a certain abnormal finding is irrelevant or even has a protective effect. For example, the absence of menstruation in a young woman can be due to a protective action that the body develops towards other problems affecting it, such as anaemia, a large weight loss, but also personal, inner problems. Considering other aspects, other data that are not always measurable, can be of enormous importance in that particular patient. We call *science* that knowledge which offers a guarantee of certainty and of its own validity, instead of that small planet of the measurable, countable and objectifiable, which remains a prisoner of the world of *opinion* and which is the antithesis of the science advocated by Aristotle and Plato.

Part I. General notions

The natural world and the spiritual world meet right from the beginning of the life of a human, in the process of fertilisation: a union is established between the bodily process represented by the germ cells, that is, by an earthly process that is transmitted from generation to generation, and the spiritual individuality that comes from a life prior to birth. The spiritual individuality connects to the living physical process, the carrier of hereditary. The first fundamental encounter between a worldly process and a spiritual process occurs here. We are used to considering the spirit-soul as something exclusively related to the sphere of the conscious, of the inner life, but it is already acting in man during his embryonic life as a powerful moulder and organizer of the body, according to the hierarchical organization of that individual. Its two fundamental components, the astral body, expression of the soul, and the organization of "I", expression of the spirit, allow us an inner life but at the same time are forces organizing the body. The embryo is not organized and modelled by the forces of hereditary alone, but is also significantly shaped by the spirit-soul forces. This explains why babies are already individuals at birth; for example, each one of two monozygotic twins[6] has a different, unique, unrepeatable personality, or history, an absolutely individual biography, because our personal history belongs to the spirit and not to nature.

At the time that a baby is born, he is already an individual because his soul and spirit have been shaping his body. This moulding action of the spirit-soul continues, albeit less strongly, lifelong. The soul continuously develops and maintains the life of our organs.

Knowing about these relationships between the spirit-soul and our organs and our bodily processes is of paramount importance, otherwise we only ever reach the extremely hazy, vague and imprecise concepts of *psychosomatic medicine*. This stems from pure

---

[6] *Monozygotic or monochorionic twins*, derived from a single fertilised egg, have identical genetic material and are supplied by the same embryonic and foetal adnexae. They are individuals who have an identical genetic code.

Health and illness

observations: in certain emotional situations, something happens in the body – the heart begins to beat strongly, an ulcer develops in the stomach, the hands become cold or the person suffers hot flushes.

Psychosomatic medicine is limited to findings: it coins nice terms and fine words, forming a smokescreen which hides absolute emptiness. Nowadays there is much trumpeting of the expression "somatisation". In reality we are all the result of somatisation. Somatisation is the process through which the spirit becomes corporeal, being immersed in space and time.

Our human shape, the capacity to stay upright in space, are expressions of the work of the spirit, of the organization of "I" on the body. In all our bodily being we are a somatisation and it is obvious that changes in our inner state are manifested by the body.

We will return to the concept of somatisation in the chapter on anxiety in the second part of this book. Anthroposophy enables a precise investigation of the relations between the spirit-soul and a given organ. For a more in-depth study of this subject, we refer the reader to the seminal works by Rudolf Steiner[7].

Here we only want to mention the relationship between the fourfold constitution of man and the conscious:

Human constitution		State of consciousness
"I"		wakefulness
ASTRAL BODY		dreaming
———————	RHYTHM	———————
ETHER BODY		sleep
PHYSICAL BODY		death

[7] Consult the catalogue of Anthrosophic Press (Steiner Books) for a list of the fundamental works by Rudolf Steiner. We would like to mention two: the first, *An Outline of Esoteric Science* (CW 13), an approach to the anthroposophic view of the world, and the second, *The Philosophy of Freedom* (CW 4), which gives this anthroposophic view a framework to understand its philosophy.

Part I. General notions

The PHYSICAL and ETHERIC whole is our living body, the one that remains in bed when we sleep, because when we wake up, the spirit-soul enters us. The ASTRAL BODY, which we can call *soul*, enters us and then the "I", the *spirit*. When we speak of sleep, we are along that line between dreaming and sleeping: there is an alternation between separation and interpenetration of the spirit-soul part and the physical-etheric part. This interplay between the astral and etheric gives rise to a *rhythm* within us, the fundamental rhythm between wakefulness and sleep.

It is precisely a disturbance in rhythm that is always the root cause of *illness*. Before an illness changes the structure of the processes of metabolism or causes damage to tissues or other symptoms, it is manifested in the rhythmic sphere. Allow me to emphasize the profundity of the anthroposophic perspective, which enables us to pick up an illness before there has been any organic effect; before any possible harm, even the most subtle, there is a change in the rhythmic play between sleep and dreaming. It was this refined diagnosis that gave rise to medicine: the priest observed the sleep of an individual, looking for any changes between sleeping and dreaming. This was the dawn of medicine[8].

It is right that, with time, the physician has been separated from the priest, but it should not be forgotten that their task is the same: working for Harmony (the physician) and for Good (the priest).

The first possible origin of illness is where the soul meets the living process. This occurs in infinite ways, but in sleeping and waking there is the rhythmic alternation between the separation and re-union of astral body and ether body. During sleep the "I" and the astral body, freed from their bond with the physical-etheric body, flow forth into their original world, the spiritual home, to

---

[8] The *incubatio* was a type of sleep induced by a priest in a temple; a reminder of this practice, which was at the origin of medicine in the western world, can be found in the word *"incubation"*, used in medicine to mean the time in which a microbe works in the body *before symptoms appear*.

Health and illness

gather more powers, and leave the physical-etheric finally free to rebuild and regenerate the vital forces of the body, in order that the bodily instrument can once again be used in its entirety. "Becoming yourself again" in the morning should be considered in the literal sense of the "I"'s renewed possession of its bodily casing. Seen as a whole, the sleep-wake rhythm is comparable to breathing on a higher plane. We can, therefore, sleep profoundly or lightly, just as we can breathe deeply or shallowly.

This conception does not contradict the changes, observed by the neurophysiologist, which occur in the cerebral cortex during sleep, but which alone cannot explain the essence of sleep. Only an expansion of knowledge and, in particular, the inclusion of the spirit-soul, resolve the important anthropological problem of sleep in its totality. The strong destructive activity in the wakeful state, which results in the drastic need for a relapse into the unconsciousness of sleep, is the prerequisite for the development of consciousness. Wherever a soul life must arise, the up-building powers of metabolism must be thwarted. For this reason, in the brain, the nerve cells even lack the capacity to reproduce and, therefore, grow in any way. During wakeful life, with the resumption of cerebral activity, there are continual processes of demolition and loss of form: the result is tiredness in the evening and the need to sleep.

We pay for the aptitude to conscious soul life and spiritual activity with a daily loss of organic life and, therefore, with a natural tendency to become ill, which is first indicated by tiredness and fatigue.

Every day of our conscious life we lose, for ever, some of our neurones. This fact provides the important information that illness does not affect us more or less randomly from the outside, but belongs to our human condition.

Illness is the price we pay for conscious life. Man is undeniably the sickest being on the planet, if you think about how often plants and animals get ill compared to humans. It is precisely this inability to pick up the peculiarity of illness in humans that prevents conventional medicine from having a scientifically valid conception of disease: it is forced to resort to a statistical criterion, according to which illness occurs whenever the data considered move away from the average.

This scientific conception verges on ideological fanaticism: when a disease is statistically more frequent than the healthy state, the disease itself becomes health; in this way we arrive at the paradox that not having dental caries means being ill and having it is a sign of health! It would then be better to be ill, that is, to deviate from the norm, and not have either caries or toothache ... We have talked about illness. But where is the healing force in man?

Centuries ago, Paracelsus already spoke of the internal healer. The most important healing process offered by nature against the illness latent in man's condition is that very state of sleep that is neither pause nor rest; for us it is an active phase of healing. Respecting the internal healer is a formidable commitment for ourselves and for those with whom we are growing, and offers a great opportunity for us to have a practical influence on our health.

I would like to mention a clinical case from over twenty years ago. One of my patients suffered from a very severe disease that is difficult to treat, ulcerative colitis. Medicine usually only tries to keep dormant this terrible chronic inflammation of the bowels, which damages the mucosa and causes numerous bleeding ulcers. Together with the patient, who was particularly trusting, we worked hard and managed to eliminate the cortisone and anti-inflammatory drugs that he had been forced to take continuously. We had not, however, managed to achieve that remission of symptoms which set his mind at rest. Finally, one evening I gave a lecture on anthroposophic medicine. I devoted a certain part of my speech to the subject of sleep as the great healer and the first medicine saying, as I still believe today, that half an hour more of sleep, particularly at the right time, has a profound effect on chronic inflammatory diseases. Well, these modest words opened my patient's eyes and he took to going to bed earlier in the evening. He improved so clearly and stably that he astonished his endoscopist at his next check-up. Although he lives four hundred

Health and illness

kilometres from my surgery he is still my patient and lives well with his disease which has been asymptomatic for many years although we both still respect and fear it. The origins of the healing powers are to be found in sleep, since during the night these powers are not disturbed by the spirit life of consciousness and can work beneficially.

When a clairvoyant looks at a sleeping body, he can see a luminous, supersensible organization of forces that exude from every part of the physical body and illuminate it. This is the *ether body* or *vital body*. This ether body is the real carrier of every process of life, growth and form and, therefore, bears the principle of unconscious up-building and re-building of the body, i.e., healing. Future understanding of the etheric world will shake the foundations of every purely mechanistic conception of life and will be the scientific basis of a natural form of farming, such as biodynamic agriculture[9]. In fact, it is the world of plants, as the first kingdom of life, that manifests the etheric-cosmic forces in the purest way and it is for this reason that this kingdom not only provides us with food, but is also a source of the curative remedies of phytotherapy. Using plant remedies, the physician can continue and promote the healing properties of the constructive etheric forces in man in a natural way. For this reason, Steiner, the founder of anthroposophic medicine, stated that true healing must involve treatment of the ether body of man.

---

[9] See: Sergio Maria Francardo, *I semi del futuro. Riflessioni di un medico sui cibi transgenici,* Edilibri, Milan 2001.

Fever and the warmth body

We would like now to consider a crucial theme in order to grasp the attitude with which anthroposophic medicine approaches illnesses, that is, the problems of fever and its meaning. The four fundamental components from which the human being is formed – a *physical body*, an *ether body*, an *astral body* and the "I"[10] or *organization of "I"* – are related to the four elements known since antiquity: earth (solid state), water (liquid state), air (gaseous state) and fire (heat or warmth). This relationship is expressed by the fact that the four constituent parts of the human being require a *medium*, a means through which they can exert their action on the human body. Here we resume schematically the relationships between the four kingdoms of nature, the physical states and the operating bodies.

KINGDOM	STATE OF MATTER	BODY
Mineral	*solid*	*physical*
Plant	*solid*	*physical*
	liquid	*ether*
Animal	*solid*	*physical*
	liquid	*ether*
	gas	*astral*
Human being	*solid*	*physical*
	liquid	*ether*
	gas	*astral*
	warmth	*"I"*

[10] The *"I"*, the spiritual part of the human being, working within the intricate reality of the body, constitutes a set of functions that, in anthroposophic medicine, we call the *Organization of "I"*. Often, for simplicity, we use the term "I" to refer to the functional aspect, to the operative vehicles that the "I" creates in the various parts of the human body. The heat body is one of these operative vehicles of the "I". In this book we often use just the word "I", for reasons of readability.

Fever and the warmth body

The regulation of body warmth is a specific activity of man's organization of "I". Without entering into too much detail, we can say that from the point of view of spiritual science, warmth is a substance, whereas from the point of view of today's physics it is an energy. We talk about the *warmth body* precisely to emphasize that it is something concrete, a real substance that acts in man. When we refer to warmth, we are not therefore discussing an energy but something that is extremely concrete.

Warmth is not, therefore, only a physical experience, but also a spirit-soul experience. It is at the origin of man's manifestation and, as can be discovered from studying anthroposophy, is also at the basis of the evolution of the Earth[11]. Man, as a spirit-soul being, carries within him a warmth that is not comparable to that of the external world; he carries within himself his own original warmth which is continuously stoked and produced by all his organs. It is precisely because he is, usually, warmer than the world that surrounds him and because he is formed of his own world of warmth, that man experiences himself as an independent being on Earth. If he were as cold as a fish, he would not be able to use the word "I" to refer to himself. This is exemplified well by children who start to use the pronoun "I" only at around the age of three years, at the conclusion of a complex process in which the child acquires a certain thermal autonomy. In fact, the temperature of a neonate exposed to the cold drops rapidly, whereas a child of three years has an intrinsic capacity to maintain his body warmth autonomously and only then can refer to himself using the word "I" and no longer impersonally as he did previously[12].

Warmth is a way for man to experience directly the action of the "I" on himself. Blood is the central element of the activity of the "I", in that it is the source of human warmth. In fact, we know that it is the blood that spreads warmth through the body. It is a

---

[11] Rudolf Steiner, *An Outline of Esoteric Science* (CW 13). In particular, the fourth chapter describes the spiritual evolution of the Earth.
[12] First he said "Baby wants food", then he will say: "I want food" (even though in my times, the prompt reply was "I want, never gets").

wonderful experience for a doctor, when he examines a patient, to try to capture the warmth of a patient, that patient's own particular warmth. This is not a romantic notion, but a real, tangible experience.

The doctor is also given precise indications from this experience of the patient's warmth. For example, when prescribing the two great anthroposophic and homeopathic remedies for febrile states, *Aconitum* and *Belladonna,* the doctor must consider the different types of warmth expressed by the patient: we advise *Aconitum* to the patient who has a much more internal warmth, more contained within the body, while we advise *Belladonna* to the patient whose warmth irradiates, whose warmth is perceived by the doctor even before he touches the patient with his own hand. Obviously, the fact that warmth irradiates depends on transpiration; a patient who is sweating irradiates more warmth to the exterior, but this external appearance simply highlights a different relationship between the organization of "I" and the astral body. We are speaking of reality, of concrete, profound physiology when we say that warmth is related to the organization of the "I".

We were talking about the doctor who examines a patient and finds different temperatures, different levels of warmth in the body, for example, an organ that is cold, or one part of the patient's body that is cooler than the rest of his body. These may be indicators that the organization of "I" has a different hold on different parts of the body; they are, therefore, important in choosing a given treatment or drug to boost the action of the "I" in a particular part of the body or in general.

The normal physical temperature of the human body is about 37 °C, a temperature that reflects the normal balance between the internal forces of warmth. If the temperature goes up, the person has a *fever*. Essentially, this means that the organization of "I" is more active within the body. In a febrile state, the "I" has to work harder than it does in normal conditions; this greater effort of the "I" enables the body to overcome illnesses more easily. After all, when we lower the temperature artificially, by taking an antipyretic such as aspirin (acetylsalicylic acid) or paracetamol, we are doing nothing other than denying the patient's "I" the possibility of entering the body more deeply, inwardly penetrating the sick body: we are counteracting the "I"'s own work. We should instead, in our attempts to cure someone, respect the work of the "I", aimed at restoring the body's original balance. In this respect a fever has an essentially positive value. This value was well recognized by the old family doctors of the past, who always had a certain respect for fever. Modern immunology is entirely consistent with this concept, having discovered that our immune system becomes more active and effective under the stimulus of a fever, while most micro-organisms become weaker and are more readily attacked by our white blood cells.

Moreover, proverbial household wisdom has handed down the opinion that when a child has a fever his body grows, he "shoots up", becoming "big". Naturally, if the fever escapes the control of the "I" it can become dangerous. For example, a rapid increase in temperature in children can cause *febrile seizures*, while a *persistent fever in an elderly person* can exhaust the patient's limited reserves, just as in the *patient weakened by chemotherapy*. I want to emphasize that fear is a poor counsellor; sometimes humble hygienic measures, such as cold compresses to the calves or a medicine such as *Belladonna* or *Aconitum*, can help the "I" in its work. I am convinced that it is almost never necessary to break a fever, thereby avoiding the consequences of doing so. Indeed, not everyone knows that too fast a decrease in temperature (febrile lysis), often caused by antipyretics, can also be a cause of seizures in childhood. From a scientific point of view it is surprising that antibiotics and antipyretics are often prescribed together, and yet it is known that fever potentiates the action of antibiotics. The patient's temperature is probably lowered to provide reassurance, to relieve anxiety, but doing so makes the illness last longer. Sometimes we have experiences that amaze us. Recently a patient of mine with a malignant tumour telephoned to tell me that a few drops of *Apis D3* and *Belladonna D4* in alternation had lowered a temperature that neither antibiotics nor antipyretics had managed to control. There are fevers that come from the metabolic pole and respond better to remedies that act on the metabolism rather than to powerful drugs that attack microbes or influence the nervous system. The day after the patient was able to face a session of chemotherapy, helped by anthroposophic medicine, and endure the complications better.

I have given this example, which is certainly outside the scope of this book, to illustrate two important points. The first is that non-conventional medicines are not always simply remedies for minor disturbances, as is often believed; the second is that no doctor and no medical doctrine is omnipotent, and if current knowledge offers an opportunity, for example chemotherapy, it could be an error to refuse it, just as it is certainly an error not to accept the help that anthroposophic medicine offers to alleviate, even if only in part, the most invasive and painful effects of chemotherapy.

The importance of nutrition to health in childhood

Introduction
Food is a live substance, not a dead one and precisely for this reason it enters into an active interplay with the forces that model the body. The first real prevention in the field of nutrition is awareness of and attention to the *quality of the food* that we eat, and this is particularly the case with regards to our children. The quality of food is a subject that has long been recognized by the more careful consumers who search for foods from healthy agriculture, which can produce wholesome products of a quality suitable for human nutrition. Furthermore, the composition and the quality of food must correspond to the nature of the human formative forces. Indeed, it is even more important to adjust the diet to a person's physical and mental states, which change in the various phases of life, such as infancy and youth. Waldorf pedagogy taught that education must respect the successive stages of development of the child and the same holds true for nutrition.
Rudolf Steiner warned that too great an intake of proteins in early childhood could predispose to the onset of sclerosis, which underlies the degenerative diseases that are the scourge of our society. It is, therefore, important to be able to choose the quality and quantity of proteins appropriate for a child's development during his growth. It is even more important that the proteins come from balanced foods, an essential precondition in order to be able to meet the complex requirements of the human "I" which gradually penetrates the body. Making the body an instrument of the developing individual means working for his freedom.

Nutritional education
A very extensive discussion would be required to address the issue of nutritional education adequately, taking into account the numerous aspects of the life and nature of children. It is a great educational issue, a pedagogy consistent with our times, which

recognizes that it has the noble task of promoting real "formation" and which ensures that the spirit and the soul of the young flourish, but which also pays attention to the formation of their body. It is an education that deems that full spirit-soul development is possible only on the foundation of a healthy physical body; a pedagogy that knows just how much the small child surrenders fully to the experiences of the external world, how much he is completely open to sensory perceptions. How can we fail to see a connection between the extraordinary acceleration in development that the sensory organs of a child undergoes under the stimulation of our modern education (intrusive sounds, bright colours, overly defined images, exciting and emotionally charged, nauseating or fake odours, artificial flavours, objects that are too perfect, leaving no possibility for development, materials that deaden the sense of touch, etc.), and the frequent diseases of the sites of the main sensory organs, located in the human head, that is, the nose, mouth and throat, ears and eyes?

This acceleration does not take into any account the principles of development in childhood and thus the family, school and sport become causes of illness. It is not the school itself that causes illness, not the profane communion of germs, nor yet sport, but the contents of these institutions which make a child ill now and which will make him an adult with weak internal organs in the future. Two crucial factors participate in the formation of the infant body: the *force of heredity* and the very *individuality of the child*. The individuality expresses the essence already present before birth (the spirit) and works ceaselessly to realise itself in the body which it has been given by the stream of heredity. Human individuality is expressed in the shape of the body.

We see the uniqueness of a person in his bearing and gait, in his facial features, in the shape of his hands, and so on. Likewise, the internal organs are imprinted by the individuality. The "I" of man must be continuously realized through the body, it must be incarnated and embodied: in doing so, it shapes the form and structure of the body. The small child does not oppose almost any of the influences from the external world, *and so these act directly as*

The importance of nutrition to health in childhood

formative impulses on the internal organs. It is for this reason that hyperstimulation translates into a forced acceleration of the child's physical and mental development, as an expression of the inability to deal with the excessive stimuli. This acceleration complicates the work of the immune system, which must clarify and understand what belongs to itself (*self*) and what does not (*not self*). The main cause of the impressive spread in allergic diseases and food intolerances is this confusion, this chaos which bewilders the immune system, provoking exaggerated, exasperated responses that are not required, and leaving undefended areas of the body that need to be protected.

Let us turn now to nutrition. What is its role in all this? It provides the substance with which, so to speak, the sculptor models his work of art, that is, the organs. The sculptor must have the right material to be able to create his work. It does, therefore, appear that the *quality of food* is of the utmost importance; good quality food is the prerequisite for a *healthy formation of the organs*. Food has nothing to do with the mechanistic idea of complex molecules that replace worn out parts of the body, but expresses the dynamics of life. Thanks to the life of which it is stripped during digestion, food enters into an active interaction with the metabolic forces of the body. Eating means passing through a disease process from which we are healed by the digestion. The most important and largest organ of the human immune system is therefore the digestive apparatus. Digestion and immune activity are two sides of the same coin.

A dynamically evolving nutrition

The composition and quality of food must also be consistent with the type of formative forces, which change depending on the age of the child. Just as education must respect the successive stages of a child's development, so too must nutrition.

The infant receives the gift of breast milk and lets its dynamic action flow almost unaltered through its body. Only after a few months will the baby start to develop his own activity towards food and only then will the child begin to be offered increasing amounts of fruit, vegetables, cereals and cow's milk. At this point food becomes an extraneous, foreign substance and must be completely demolished. Starting from this period the substance of the body is created from scratch, but the activity of the newly created body is influenced by the fundamental vital structure of the food: the up-building is oriented by the stimuli.

There are two possible basic errors of nutrition:
– in the first, the stimulus is too weak: we have *undernutrition*;
– in the second, in contrast, the foreign vital forces are too strong and impose part of their being on the child's formative forces: in this case we have *overnutrition*.

In the latter case the organs become too large and the spiritual individuality of the child cannot penetrate the body's substrate sufficiently. The former condition is widespread in the Third World, while the latter threatens children in areas of material well-being in industrialised countries. This is not simply a question of overeating: on the one hand the forces of the child's body are engaged beyond measure, and on the other their needs are not met. In this sense, there is an undernutrition in all this abundance. The table is laden, but the children are starving.

In which foods is the extraneous life force too strong? What type of mistaken diet can lead to organic structures that are too compact, in which the "I" has difficulty in manifesting itself?

Protein overloading

The intake of protein is exaggerated these days. Just consider that in some situations modern paediatricians and nutritionists, who often give bewildering and distorted information, are not consistent with the basic principles that they themselves set out.

For example, it is thought that the correct protein intake is little more than one gram of protein per kilogram of body weight. This amount – which could be debated since it does not take into account the quality of the proteins or correct associations between foods, which allow substantial protein saving while adapting the diet to the greater protein requirements of children – is vastly exceeded in infancy. Just consider that a simple yoghurt portion weighing 125 grams contains 5 grams of protein: this means that a child weighing ten kilograms (the average weight at about the age of one year) has already met his daily protein requirement with only two and a half yoghurts!

It would be counterproductive for advertising to vaunt the protein value of a snack if doctors, educators and parents were informed correctly, because it becomes difficult not to exceed the protein needs of the body when eating such snacks. You can easily verify that the protein supply is continuously in excess of needs in the diets that are advised nowadays.

I recently saw a four-year old girl I had examined for the first time a few months previously. During that first examination the little girl was feverish and filled the waste basket in my surgery with paper tissues soaked with phlegm. She had suffered from colds with catarrh uninterruptedly since she was six months old, snored at night because of her huge adenoids and was always getting sick. In her third year of life she had been prescribed ten courses of antibiotics for a total of more than seventy days of treatment; that is, one day in every five she was under antibiotic therapy.

Having arrived in this state, I prescribed her a diet based on alternating biodynamic wholemeal cereals, biological or biodynamic olive oil, fundamental vegetables such as biodynamic carrots, fennel and beetroot, for fruit only biodynamic apples and pears, biological bread and spelt wheat biscuits, a few almonds and hazelnuts, biodynamic flavouring (dried or fresh when possible) on all food and, as a snack, biological carrot juice or a few biological biscuits.

I asked the mother for an act of faith, advising her to let herself be helped by her sister who has been a patient of mine for a long time and is an expert at cooking wholemeal grains. The result: the girl has not been ill in the last eight months! Not even once. Her vulva, which was as red as a pepper because of the accumulation of preservatives and colourants is now pinkish, the child sleeps peacefully and is much calmer.

Her teachers at the nursery school asked the mother whether the child was taking sedatives[13], because she had become calm and collaborative. The mother was astonished by the results obtained and asked why I didn't spread this information. I replied that I had been doing so for almost thirty years.

I had to explain to this mother that even in Waldorf schools there has been, and there still is, strong pressure to give already overfed children ham, ice-cream and puddings. The acrid odour of their limbs and the redness of the rims of their eyes, an effect of food preservatives, are unequivocal signs of over-nutrition; these signs are often associated with intoxication by phosphorus and proteins, which blocks their fantasy, suffocated by a clogged metabolism. In the past, immoral generals ordered that their troops be given phosphorus-based preparations to render them aggressive and ruthless. Nowadays, what do we give to these children who can't stay still for a minute? They live between one crisis of abstinence and another, and so they scream to have their snack until their parents give in.

The child's meal is prepared according to a menu for an adult. We are raising little gourmets. "Darling, what would you like today? Chicken breast with asparagus or beef in tomato sauce?", asks a modern mother, unjustly making her child responsible for choices that rightly belong to the parent. The youngsters grow, apparently flourishing, seem solid, bursting with energy and dynamism and look at the world with interest. The observer is tricked into believing in the merits of an early diet of meat.

Of course, a distinction must be made between the proteins of animal origin: while *meat* and *fish* are substances from the body of animals, a whole animal will be born from an *egg*. Thus the proteins of an egg develop great dynamism and strongly stimulate growth. In contrast, the proteins of *milk*, which is not part of an animal, but a substance destined to feed growing animals, are

---

[13] You will certainly know that psychotropic medicines, drugs similar to amphetamines, are being used to "treat" agitated, difficult children who have the so-called "attention deficit disorder"; prescriptions have increased vertiginously in the United States in recent years. We have even reached the point that children are now prescribed antidepressants, such as the famous Prozac.

particularly suitable for children, if given in reasonable amounts. Meat, containing proteins from an adult animal, conveys the already weighty, completely mature "being". The use of suckling calves arose precisely from the need to mitigate this effect, by using a young animal that has been fed only milk. Through the early introduction of a diet based on meat, eggs and fish, we are promoting the development of a compact body that nevertheless masks the formation of a coarse bodily structure that is only apparently robust and that cannot be fully grasped and penetrated by the person's "I". The "I" is prevented from being able to build up its bodily instrument in such a way that it can work freely. The organic structure of a body that is not entirely worked through by the "I" will not have sufficient reactive capacities, thus laying the basis for *sclerosis*. The formation of a bodily substance that can be moulded and penetrated correctly by the "I" is determined by the quality of the food from which we derive the proteins for our nourishment. Just as it is critical to choose the proteins appropriate for the child's stage of development, so too is it important that these proteins are obtained from balanced foods such as biodynamic products, which stand out by a remarkable vital dynamism that satisfies the complex needs of the human "I".

Surplus proteins favour sclerosis because they allow hypermineralisation, since minerals (for example, iron) bind to proteins.

Another consequence of excess proteins, particularly animal proteins that are not completely dominated by the body, is a toxic effect produced by the undigested protein residues. Such excesses of not completely dominated vital processes modify the relationship with micro-organisms which proliferate thanks to this overflowing of vital processes. The result is an alteration in our bacterial flora and the body, in our very intestines, the biggest organ of our immune defence system, becomes the object of a life alien to its original forces. Micro-organisms feed on this extraneous life which, not having been dominated entirely by the digestive process, is still the life of the animals from which the proteins were derived. *A surplus of proteins, therefore, increases the predisposition to infectious diseases.*

The tendency to produce catarrh, so widespread nowadays, represents an important reaction of the body aimed at counteracting the tendency to hardening, "sclerosis", a manifestation of the extraneous life that is deposited. This reaction is an attempt to restore malleability to a body that is hardening and tries, through this centrifugal process (expulsive action), to expel this parasitic life from within the body to its exterior.

Independently of the "mad cow" problem and the presence of hormones and antibiotics in animal foods, we can say that *reducing protein intake, particularly proteins of animal origin, is a good defence against catarrh and infections.*

Many mothers of children who have been switched to an almost vegetarian diet have seen, often very clearly, a notable reduction in recurrent episodes of catarrhal infections, which decrease considerably as surplus protein is eliminated and protein of direct animal origin is withdrawn. There is no need to fear protein deficiency with a proper wholemeal diet, since the various cereals are alternated and associated with seasonal vegetables, fruit, seeds and pulses. The cereals should preferably be grown biodynamically. In fact, the formation of proteins is disturbed by the forced fertilisation of industrial farming and certain illnesses in children are due precisely to this phenomenon.

This same consideration also holds true for the precious formation of protein in green leaves. Dr. Renzenbrink, an anthroposophic nutritionist, gave a clear example: incomplete maturation of proteins in spinach gives rise to toxic intermediate products. This caused cases of severe poisoning of babies in Germany, such that paediatricians advised mothers not to give their children spinach to eat in the first few years of life. The quantity of undesired nitrates in spinach can range from 59 to 1872 milligrams per kilogram; in carrots, the most precious vegetable for children, it ranges from 2 to 2235 milligrams per kilogram, while the amount of lead in carrots varies from 0 to 359 milligrams per kilogram.

The warning against the consumption of spinach would not be necessary if we were to use biodynamic products, provided that the spinach is harvested at the right time and not too early. There

The importance of nutrition to health in childhood

is no worse spinach than frozen spinach, harvested prematurely for understandable but not healthy commercial reasons. However, grown correctly, this vegetable has the highest nutritional value for a child and can play a useful role in the child's diet. In general, we should try to avoid cooked and frozen foods that advertising suggests we fry in oil totally lacking in any nutritional value.

Flavouring foods to help the immune system
Another important principle is to include aromatic herbs gradually into the child's diet.
We can already use such herbs during breastfeeding, when we prescribe the mother a herbal tea based on Umbelliferae, such as a *tisane of cumin* (fennel, anise, cumin), which has the dual effect of increasing the production of breast milk and promoting the neonate's digestion. Subsequently, we can give the aromas and spices directly in the child's food. Aromas also help the healthy individual, because they arouse impulses that are apparently modest but that influence nutrition beneficially.
A soup that is lightly flavoured, for example by adding cumin seeds, is useful for involving the whole body in the uptake and processing of the food and for providing warmth for the metabolism without stressing it. Supplying warmth through the administration of cumin or a drink of vodka has enormously different effects on the body's forces, as we can readily understand from the following example: we can imagine developing warmth as a result of a good run (complete digestion produces warmth, just as does running) or by turning on the heating (we are passive and, in essence, weakened). Furthermore, it has been shown that both salivary flow and the enzymes within the saliva are potentiated by the intake of spicy foods.
Hot spices stimulate the gastric juices and help, in particular, the digestion of proteins, which is useful given that poor digestion of proteins promotes the formation of phlegm. Other spices activate the digestive glands (liver, gallbladder, pancreas) directly, thereby promoting the secretion of their juices in the intestines.
Thanks to an improved digestion, it also becomes easier for the

body to assimilate other food and build up new human substance entirely worked through by our most inner and complex part, by our organization of "I". This new substance does not require other "rearranging" to be made suitable for constituting the human being. Our metabolic centre does not, therefore, need to reprocess the substances and expel them in the form of phlegm, as it presently does for inappropriately high protein foods. As far as regards flavouring, it is better to use biodynamic products, or at least certified "biological" herbs and spices. In fact, most flavourings produced by intensive cultivation contain large amounts of pollutants and are irradiated and sterilised with gamma rays, the same rays that are claimed to be harmless by industry and are used to sterilise syringes and colour laboratory glass yellow. Many foods contain precious amounts of silicon, which is essential for the skin, mucous membranes, nails, hair and connective tissue. Silicon is the substance used to make glass, and when irradiated with gamma rays becomes yellow. Would it not perhaps be prudent to avoid food and flavours containing silicon that have been tainted by radiation? You may have noticed that industrial flavours are like laboratory glass that does not let light pass through: they have no life and remain for ever on the shelves without ever ageing. It is always better to be suspicious of food that does not perish and that never goes bad. For the same reasons, excessive use of white sugar is not recommended, since this is no longer part of a plant, but a crystal.

An object has value over time if it has the intrinsic possibility to express the human use for which it was made: a wooden table ages and acquires value, whereas a table made of Formica remains identical and loses value. Just as the hand of a child who touches Formica is deprived of a tactile experience related to the recognition of the work of time, so too is it important for our mucosal membranes to perceive time in the life of food, to feel that one apple has just been picked from a branch and still smells of the forces of heaven, whereas another has long been in a basket and its taste gives the sensation of over-ripeness.

We do not want food as perfect as a machine, but genuine food!

Healthy choices and healthy habits: the central role of biodynamic wholemeal cereals

Basically, we want to say that health, undoubtedly determined by numerous, complex factors, can be positively influenced by some correct nutritional measures, which are particularly important in childhood: avoid overnutrition and food that is too "far" from nature, introduce foods into the diet gradually, and respect the annual rhythm of nature as well as environmental conditions and the weather. For example, the year-round availability of a summer food, such as chili pepper, is a real dietary error; a pepper's capacity to dissipate warmth does not make it suitable for a winter day. Furthermore, we should avoid early intake of animal proteins, use few dairy products and eat biological pulses. The various wholemeal cereals, essential seasonal vegetables and high quality, biodynamic fruit should be the core of the diet. It is also important to use spices and herbs in the food, particularly in the autumn before the start of catarrhal illnesses. Spices are excellent food preservatives outside the body, and in the past have saved whole populations without refrigerators from starvation, but once inside the body they work in the opposite way from chemical preservatives, facilitating the recognition of the foods by the digestive system and thereby helping the digestion. In this way they can reduce those allergies and food intolerances that are affecting us ever more frequently.

I would like to recall the various *biodynamic wholemeal cereals* as dietary "testimonials" of universalism and of cosmopolitanism, because every cereal expresses a culture of human history, from the *millet* of the Africans – the precious cradle of mankind – to the *corn* of the magical native populations of America. The variety of healthy wholemeal cereals has an educative effect on our metabolism: we need different stimuli derived from beings that are related but as widely different as the grasses, just as in thought we need different human cultures in order to be free men.

In this sense, an ancient grain such as spelt expresses the essence of Romanity which brought order and a drive towards reciprocal integration between different cultures and populations; the effort required to digest such an intricate grain helps to bring order to the intestinal flora and, if I may say, leads to a healthy and essential coexistence with our bacterial friends.

Let's turn now to the richness of the very healthy fats contained in the wonderful sesame seed[14], with a protein content that works so well with a diet based on wholemeal cereals. Note that durum flour Sicilian bread contains sesame seeds, which can be used lightly toasted and possibly partially crushed to dress, flavour and enrich vegetables and cereals. Finally, nougat based on sesame seeds and honey is an authentic wonder!

These are the precious little gifts that make our diet simple, harmonious and pleasant. A sesame seed is a real treasure box of nutritional qualities, from precious fats to proteins, important for replacing deficient amino acids[15].

The poor quality fats present in all food that is pre-cooked, preserved or sold in fast-food outlets, combined with the emotional stresses of our city lives, predispose to sclerotic diseases, from the most common tumours such as bowel cancer and breast cancer, to cardiovascular disease, which is the leading cause of death in the "outsized" humans of our current, greedy era. We do, however, have the chance to remedy the situation by using very high quality fats. Open Sesame!

---

[14] Sesame paste, called "tahini", is a valuable food, useful for dressing vegetables, making cooked fruit delicious, and adding flavour to honey spread on black bread.

[15] Amino acids are the basic constituents of proteins. A healthy protein balance is not obtained from enormous amounts of protein, because this overloads the metabolism with nitrogen substances which pollute the body and underlie degenerative diseases. The best possibility of finding a balance is through a correct combination of high quality foods. For example, biodynamic wholemeal cereals, which are the foundation of a healthy diet, can be supplemented with some foods that incorporate the range of amino acids, such as pulses, eggs, small quantities of dairy products, sesame seeds and nuts (walnuts, hazelnuts and almonds); in this way we create the possibility and the opportunity to introduce balanced proteins into our body, without overloading it. The diet must be varied, but there is no need to be dazzled by supermarket shelves. Just think of bread and how many opportunities nature offers to enrich it with marvellous seeds of every type: sunflower, cumin, flax, poppy and, of course, sesame seeds.

PART TWO

Illnesses and remedies

How to deal with a fever

The first fundamental part of managing a fever is *bed rest*: the "I" needs to be relieved of its work in maintaining an upright position in order that it can be dedicated to overcoming the disease. Bed rest is very important in the treatment of viral infections, which account for the majority of the most common febrile illnesses: in the absence of bed rest, healing can be delayed and, more importantly, complications may develop. The persistent cough and colds that affect many children after a viral infection, or that torment adults, are usually the result of insufficient rest during the period of the acute infection.

Antipyretic drugs give immediate relief, but precisely for this reason, harassed adults and modern children get out of bed before being healed and, consequently, their illnesses last longer. This is why antipyretics should be used very prudently.

Right from earliest infancy, children should be convinced that they must stay in bed if they have a fever, that they should try to respect the self-healing powers of the body, which work best during rest. In this way we will rear wise adults who are aware of the damage caused by the haste that actually slows our self-healing forces and leaves us troubled.

It is also important to *hydrate the body*, because we sweat in response to an increase in temperature; if, however, we lose too much water because of a high fever, the body is forced to block the excretory ducts to limit the losses, making it difficult to deal with the fever. All that needs to be done is to *drink: water, but also pressed or squeezed fruit juice without sugar, or vegetable juices*, which are rich in mineral salts (that support the "I") and vitamins (that support the ether body, our life force).

Herb teas, such as those produced from *lime blossom* or *black elder flowers*, are also very useful: both provide fluids and salts and stimulate sweating. A tea of lime blossom sweetened with honey is recommended for children, whereas a tea of black elder flowers, or a mixture of both flowers, is preferable for adults.

One useful formula for tackling a fever is a mixture of *thyme, lime blossom, black elder flowers* and *chamomile flowers*, in equal parts[16]. This mixture combines the property of stimulating sweating, which has already been described, together with the antiseptic properties of thyme and the anti-inflammatory effects of chamomile.

All that needs to be done is to add a heaped teaspoon of the mixture into a cupful of boiling water, boil for thirty seconds and then leave the herb tea covered for ten minutes before straining it and sweetening it, as desired, with honey.

For adults

If the temperature tends to exceed 40°C, the patient can take a bath in water that is about 2°C lower than his or her rectal temperature. Before the bath it is useful to administer 10-15 drops of *Onopordon-Primula comp.* to support the circulation and to avoid complications due to the vasodilation that is caused by immersion in a fluid that is in any case warmer than the environment. People with low blood pressure, dizziness or a tendency to fainting should not take hot baths. The patient should be watched and absolutely must not take a bath alone! If the patient becomes pale, he must be helped out of the bath immediately and his body rubbed energetically with *Spirit of Melissa* or, in the absence of this, with *eau de cologne*.

---

[16] It is worth keeping a stock of the fundamental plants cited in this book, such as *thyme, chamomile, lime, elder,* and *sage*. It is important that the plants are of *biodynamic quality*, which can be determined from the trademarks *Demeter* (a mark of consolidated biodynamics) and *Byodin* (a quality label of transitional biodynamic agriculture). If these cannot be obtained, look for herbs of organic quality or collections of wild plants. With the spread of herbalism and the interest in 'returning to nature', the market has grown in an exponential manner but, unfortunately, some of the herb teas sold are heavily polluted. I am sorry to say it, but many of the herbs come from intensive farming with massive use of weed-killers, pesticides and synthetic fertilisers. In contrast, the companies connected to anthroposophic and homeopathic medicine use herbs of known quality and, in particular, those with an anthroposophic leaning, privilege biodynamic or wild products.

A basic remedy for a fever is *Bryonia/Eucalyptus comp*. The dose is 10-12 drops in a little water every one or two hours, depending on the intensity of the fever. Once an improvement has obtained, the frequency of the treatment should be reduced gradually to accompany the healing, rather than abruptly withdrawing it.

For children
A very important remedy for controlling a rapidly rising temperature or an already high one (above 39°C) is *damp compresses applied to the feet and calves*. These are prepared by putting some water at room temperature, or better still, lukewarm, in a bowl and adding lemon juice or a couple of teaspoons of vinegar in order to promote evaporation. Pieces of cotton or linen are soaked in this liquid, wrapped round the child's feet and calves, and then covered with terry towels.

An adult's woollen socks are another very practical way to cover compresses. The child's warmth will dry the pieces of cloth, which can then be soaked again. This very simple remedy has the advantages of protecting the child from the risks of a high temperature and of giving the nervous system some relief. These compresses are much less unpleasant than an bag of ice on the head and do not risk cooling the part of the body where the infection is, given that fevers in children are often caused by illnesses that involve precisely the head.

Furthermore, anthroposophic medicine teaches that there is an important relationship between the head and feet: for example, a good warm foot bath can relieve a catarrhal disease of the head. The headaches that affect a febrile child are often due to a particular type of sinusitis (ethmoiditis) which frequently goes undiagnosed; it is not a good idea to aggravate any disease by applying an ice pack.

The compresses do not lower the body temperature drastically, but do slow its rise and are always well tolerated. Personally, I prefer lemon juice to vinegar, because it seems more pleasant to me.

Another measure that is always useful in children, but also in adults, is an *enema*: it has hydrating and decongestant effects and also lowers the temperature slightly. We will talk about this remedy again in the chapter on cold-related illnesses.

A basic remedy suitable for children is *Ferrum phosphoricum comp.* From one to five globules are dissolved in the mouth every two hours. Two globules are sufficient for a child of two to three years old. This treatment should not be stopped abruptly, but continued for two or three days gradually reducing its frequency. It is, of course, useful to combine this remedy with a lime blossom tea and, possibly with compresses and an enema, if the fever is high.

Young babies can be given 7-10 globules of *Ferrum phosphoricum comp.* dissolved in three fingers of water: a teaspoonful of the preparation is given every hour. If the illness is mild and the baby is being breastfed, it may be useful to give the granules to the mother – 10 granules every one to two hours – in order that the baby receives the medication in the breast milk.

A tea of lime blossom and chamomile flowers, sweetened with a little organic raw cane sugar, can also be given in a baby's bottle. I do not advise honey for babies under the age of one year because, being a sugar that comes from flowers, it stimulates the metabolism too much and, as used to be said, it "warms" the person; it is also a laxative and inflames mucous membranes. For this reason, the habit of sweetening a baby's dummy with honey should be strongly discouraged.

Another remedy to keep in the home is *Belladonna D30*; the dose for very high fevers is from 3 to 10 drops every hour, or even every half hour if the temperature is rising rapidly with the risk of causing febrile seizures. The baby appears miserable with a flushed face and emanates heat through marked sweating; he does not want to be touched, but there are no other clinical signs. *Belladonna D30* is also strongly indicated if the child is ranting or having hallucinations.

An effective remedy in the case of a very fast developing nocturnal fever, which wakes the baby, distressing and scaring him, is *Aconitum D30* in drops or granules: 3 granules or 5-10 drops every three to four hours given a few times. The important indication for this treatment is that the child caught a cold, was exposed to the wind and/or got wet a few hours previously. *Aconitum* is another medication to keep in the house, because its effectiveness depends on it being administered promptly. If given quickly, it can ensure a rapid cure and, above all, protect against the onset of severe illnesses that can develop as result of strong exposure to cold.

Colds and cold-related illnesses

We all know the symptoms of cold-related illnesses, which occur when a foreign cold penetrates our functional organization and the body fights to restore harmony within our warmth body. We must support our body in its work of expelling *foreign cold* and "*humanising*" the cold that has worked its way into the body's structure, in order to prevent the illness from worsening.

An excellent remedy in the initial stage is a *footbath of increasing temperature*, from tepid to very hot, which makes use of the important functional relationship in the warmth body between the feet and the head: by acting on the feet, we can cause a reaction in the head, which is not an effect from "outside", but from within the body. If we want to increase the effect of this heat we can add a few teaspoons of *powdered ginger* or better still, *grated ginger root*, or, as we all know, two good handfuls of *coarse sea salt*: in fact the SAL of alchemy[17] is related to the upper pole of the human being, the head. Interestingly, the Latin word "*sal*" means both "salt" and "wit".

There is another much more effective therapy, which *must be prescribed by a doctor*[18]: the *mustard footbath*. This type of footbath has very intense effects in the region of the head and maxillary sinuses, which are often involved in more acute colds. The pain of sinusitis can be alleviated using this therapeutic measure alone. It is, however, important that the footbath does not go higher than

---

[17] Anthroposophy identifies the action of the great universal principles of alchemy in the organization of humans, thus creating the opportunity to understand the relationship between man and nature. This provides the basis for acting on an organ or its function from various points of the body:
SAL in the *head* (nerve-sense system);
MERCUR in the *centre of man* (cardiovascular and respiratory system);
SULPHUR in the *lower man* (metabolic system and limbs).

[18] We discuss treatments and remedies which must be prescribed, such as mustard footbaths, with the aim of helping patients to follow the prescriptions of their anthroposophic doctor or pharmacist, which is, after all, the purpose of this book.

the ankles, since this would provide too strong an effect on the circulation. This treatment is *strongly contraindicated in people with venous problems*, so each case must be evaluated carefully.

The footbath is prepared by putting a small amount of water in a bowl and then continuously replacing it with ever hotter water up to the level of tolerance and until the foot becomes red. The effect can be intensified by adding a few tablespoons of mustard powder and prolonging the bath for 15 minutes. The footbath has its effect when the patient has an outbreak of sweating; for this reason it is a good idea that the patient wraps himself in a blanket or bathrobe. This method can be used to treat a violent cold, sinusitis and also headaches. It can also nip an incipient cold in the bud.

A mustard footbath is strongly contraindicated during or around the period of menstruation, since it could provoke a real haemorrhage. Mustard, which is prescribed by a doctor, is usually *contraindicated in pale-skinned people, blondes and red-heads*, because these individuals can have violent reactions. The action of mustard on the skin can be likened to the effect of exposing the skin to sun: *it is better that people who have excessive reactions to the sun use remedies that do not involve mustard.*

One method, which we have already mentioned, for activating the warmth body is a *lime blossom tea*. Known for its sudorific (sweat-inducing) action, this can be considered a fundamental herbal tea for combatting various cold-related illnesses. However, a few details should be discussed. The first is that this tea is indicated only if taken by someone already in bed or just about to go to bed; if this is not the case, there is the risk of exacerbating the illness, because drinking the *lime blossom* tea, sweating and then going outdoors – perhaps even going for a ride on a moped! – creates the risk of converting an incipient cold into a full-blown pneumonia. The second point is that only the *flowers* should be used, not the *flowers and bracts* together, in order to best exploit the functional relationship between the flower of a plant[19] and

---

[19] The site of *sulphur* in plants is in its flowers, *mercur* is present in the leaves

the human metabolic system. The third detail concerns the preparation of the tea, which should be done as follows: pour a heaped teaspoonful of lime blossom into boiling water, then add two fingers of cold water to stop the boiling and wait, with the heat on, those few seconds necessary for the water to start boiling again. In this way we extract the maximum of the vital (ether) forces of the flower, whose release is favoured by the rapid change in temperature, without damaging the delicate essential oils. You can add *honey* or strengthen the tea with *black elder flowers*, another important sudorific.

The basis of the treatment of a cold is essentially good life style, although some remedies can be used.

Sambucus comp. (Sambucus D3, Berberis D6, Phosphorus D6, Teucrium scorodoniae D4) drops: this is a good remedy for colds, particularly those catarrhal forms with night sweats, irritable cough and a tendency to spread to the lower respiratory tract. The dose is 10 drops every two or three hours.

Sambucus also has a liquifying effect and soothes irritation of the rhinopharyngeal mucosae.

This remedy can also be used in children, at a dose of 3-7 drops, depending on the child's age, every two or three hours.

Another useful remedy, to combine with the lime blossom tea, is the simple *Ferrum phosphoricum comp. granules*. If the cold develops after being exposed to lower temperatures or getting wet, or in the first phase of an influenza, it is worth making generous use of this remedy: the dose is 12-15 granules every hour for adults and 2-4 granules every two hours for children. The granules should be dissolved in the mouth. Of course, children, who greatly appreciate this remedy, will chew them, but this does not

---

and *sal* in the roots. This is one of the reasons linking the parts of a plant to humans and also explains the particular care that the anthroposophic range of remedies has in using a given part of a plant. It is not the same thing to use *Chamomilla planta tota,* the whole chamomile plant, or use *Chamomilla radix*, the roots. For example, chamomile root is very useful for helping babies to cut teeth, while the *planta tota* is not specific for this indication. *I advise to comply scrupulously with the prescriptions from your anthroposophic doctor or pharmacist.*

matter, since the granules will work anyway. This remedy is very useful when the cold is the first symptom of an influenza; conceived in particular for *childhood influenza*, it also has a good effect on colds in us sickly city-dwellers, because iron and phosphorus give the nervous system a certain support. There are also two classical homeopathic remedies that are loyal helpers.

The first, *Euphrasia D3 drops*, is a remedy for colds with watery nasal discharges, which are not irritating, but with irritating ocular symptoms such as red, itchy, watery eyes. The other remedy, *Cepa D3 drops,* is useful for acute rhinitis with a marked nasal discharge that irritates and reddens the skin around the nose and the upper lip and causes frequent, violent sneezing. *Cepa D3* can be used with complete safety even in people with a recent cold who have such redness in these areas that they seem to have burnt themselves.

These two remedies are both taken in drop form, with the dose being 10 drops every one, two or three hours. *Cepa* is an onion, which is also an excellent remedy used in its natural state; for example, through their sulphurous vapours, slices of raw onion put on a plate at a child's bedside reduce swelling of the mucous membranes.

One treatment that I mention, because I used to prescribe it regularly in the past, is as follows: chop a raw onion finely and put the pieces into a thin gauze, stitch the gauze closed with sewing thread and put the bundle into the nose, pushing it backwards, not upwards, and leaving the thread hanging out in order to be able to extract the gauze. It is difficult to prescribe such remedies nowadays: they are effective, but not very suitable for us fragile contemporaries. I readily confess that the only patients I dare advise such a treatment, for themselves, are housewives, the "warriors" of today.

Another remedy is *Berberis fructus D2 drops*, a useful treatment in the case of marked inflammation and swelling of the mucosal membranes, with difficulty in secreting and a tendency for symptoms to persist. These drops are also useful for the treatment of sinusitis. Use 10 drops every two or three hours. This remedy can be given for long periods in the case of chronic rhinitis, although always under the supervision of a doctor.

If the inflammation does not recede and invades the posterior part of the nose and rhinopharynx (the upper part of the throat), while waiting to see the doctor, we can use a preparation such as *Cinnabar D20*, a tablet to dissolve in the mouth every three hours. *Cinnabar* is an ore of mercury and sulphur, a remedy which combines the typical liquifying and loosening effects of mercury with the anti-inflammatory action of sulphur. As Hippocrates taught: where there is stagnation, we must loosen and dissolve.

Inhalations and *simple steam treatments* can be useful: put the head, covered by a towel, over a bowl filled with a chamomile or thyme tea, or a litre of boiling water to which 5-10 drops of thyme essential oil have been added.

Never use essential oils with an aerosol, because they are too irritant!

I shall not dwell too much on this problem, but certainly many of the continual colds from which we suffer are the result of bad habits in protecting ourselves from the cold, in what we eat and in our daily hygiene.

Just as it is important to wrap up adequately, so too is it important to eat foods that support the warmth body, starting from the metabolism. From this point of view, biodynamic wholemeal cereals and spices are a real blessing. We must avoid foods that cause dissipation of heat, such as summer foods and foods from tropical countries. Eating a chili in winter is like unbuttoning an overcoat in a snowfall; drinking a cold beverage, full of preservatives that slow our metabolism, is like putting your hat on when you are already outside, after having filled it with cold air.

Please forgive me if I confess my distress when I see a child in the street in the middle of autumn drinking a can of cold tea or licking an ice-cream, and even more so when I realise that the child is coming through the door of my surgery.

An ice-cream a day in the cold season, washed down with a glass of industrially manufactured tea, is are the ideal way of producing lots of catarrh and weakening the immune system.

Influenza

The word "influenza" derives from the Latin *influentia*, a term which reflects the belief that epidemics of this disease are closely related to the "influence" of particularly unfavourable planetary conjunctions. On the advice of Rudolf Steiner, we anthroposophic doctors observe the movements of the planets during the course of the year with interest, but without any misplaced fanaticism. In particular, the astronomical relationship between the Sun and some of the more distant planets of the solar system (Saturn, Jupiter, Mars) confirms that some conjunctions play a role in facilitating the spread of the epidemic, reducing the magnitude of the Sun's curative effect. Obviously we listen carefully to the predictions of epidemiologists, but we also make use of this little help from the cosmos to understand the most critical periods.

For anthroposophic medicine influenza has always been a disease to take care of, whether it occurs in children or adults, In fact, influenza is an illness that has the particular characteristic of paving the way for the development of more serious diseases. I do not intend to talk only about the complications of the viral infection itself, but rather the consequences that can be manifested in the long term, years or even decades after the infection. I would like to give an example. One of the greatest epidemics of influenza in the history of mankind was the so-called "Spanish 'flu" of 1918, the most deadly epidemic known since the "Black Death" plague in the Middle Ages.

Not only was there a high death rate during the spread of the disease itself, but decades later its consequences were still being seen; there is a strong suspicion that in some elderly patients with Parkinson's disease, the Spanish 'flu played a role in activating the neurological disorder.

The famous book *Awakenings* by the neuropsychiatrist Oliver Sacks, and the touching film of the same name starring Robin Williams, recounts the story of the survivors of an epidemic of "lethargic encephalitis" connected to influenza, which spread

Influenza

through the world in the years 1917-1927, killing almost five million people. This epidemic disappeared suddenly and mysteriously, leaving a minute fraction of survivors in a sort of perpetual stupor, an "everlasting spell". Dr. Sacks administered L-dopa, a drug used to treat Parkinson's disease, to all the patients with encephalitis in a whole ward, eliciting their emotional but temporary awakening.
According to Sacks and other researchers, the influenza virus probably opened the way to the epidemic of encephalitis and potentiated the effects of the encephalitis itself.
The fact remains that between October 1918 and January 1919, when there was the terrifying pandemic of Spanish 'flu with over 21 million deaths, encephalitis appeared in a more virulent form. It is important to appreciate that in the period preceding the full-blown illness, the patient experiences a reduction in cerebral activity delegated to processing perceptions: symptomatically there is a sort of *dulling of the sensorium* from which the disease process can spread through the whole body, involving its various parts.
I hope I have convinced the reader that influenza is a disease that should be treated. Let us see how.
Bed rest. The first important measure to take is bed rest: in fact, we have to avoid tiring our nervous system and, above all, the senses, which are the first part of the body affected by the disease.
Do not overstimulate the metabolism. As said above, the origin of the disease lies in the nerves and senses; we must not, therefore, engage the metabolism in too much effort by an excessively nutrient diet in order not to drain strength from the nervous system. It is, therefore, important to pay attention to any slowing down or stoppage of bowel function. Cooked fruit is an excellent way of avoiding sudden attacks of constipation that impair the defensive activities of the intestinal immune system.
Stimulate sweating. We all know the benefit of a good sweat when we have influenza; it activates our warmth body: a sort of artificial fever is created, thanks to which, the organization of "I", which lives in the warmth, can regain control of the situation.

Part II. Illnesses and remedies

A *tea of lime blossom* or of *black elder flowers* is obviously a fundamental treatment for influenza, because these herbal teas stimulate the metabolism and sweating, thereby helping to expel the disease.
The tea, which should be drunk very hot, can initially cause an increase in body temperature, which should not cause alarm because it precedes the start of sweating. The only limitation is in small children with a very high temperature. In this case it is better to administer a less concentrated, lukewarm herb tea. As we have already said for all cold-related diseases, a tea of lime blossom is an excellent way to prevent influenza. In people, particularly children, who are susceptible to frequent infections, it should be drunk, before going to bed, for a few weeks in the period of the epidemic.
Another very useful remedy after having caught a cold or got wet is a general whole body compress, but only if the patient is in a condition to develop an adequate reaction. This treatment is not, therefore, indicated for weak or debilitated individuals, who suffer from hypotension (low blood pressure) or anaemia.
If the patient's condition does allow it, this compress, which is applied to the whole body with water or particular oils (for example, *lavender oil*), also has great benefits in the treatment of chronic diseases.
The procedure for acute illnesses, in particular for influenza, is as follows. Lay out one or two woollen blankets that extend at least 50 centimetres beyond the patient's feet and that are large enough to wrap the patient in completely. Put a smaller towel, soaked in cold water and then well wrung, on top of the blankets.
The patient should lie down, completely naked, on the cold towel, before being sponged quickly with tepid water and vinegar to set off the sweating more quickly. It is important to prepare everything necessary before starting the treatment, in order to be able to act without haste, but with a certain speed. The patient, lying on the cold, wet towel, must hold his hands crossed on his chest, so as not to feel suffocated by being too tightly bound; the towel is then closed around the patient, making it adhere per-

fectly to the body up to the level of the neck (there is a very unpleasant sensation if air gets in). Next the woollen blanket is wrapped around the patient and then hot water bottles are placed above and around the patient who is also covered with a duvet. This treatment provokes intense sweating in a short time and the person looking after the patient must dry the dripping sweat, which can be very abundant. The patient is left in this way for an hour or an hour and a half, being given a tea of lime blossom or black elder flowers to promote even more sweating. The patient emerges from this treatment as if reborn, experiencing what is a real process of healing and feeling cleansed within. If possible this treatment should be carried out on a double bed, because at the end of the established time, the procedure is to extract first one arm from the wrapping, rapidly sponge it with lukewarm water, dry the arm and then slip it into the sleeve of a pyjama top before putting it under a dry blanket; next, the other arm is extracted, sponged, dried, sleeved and put under the dry blanket, and so on, washing and drying the patient a little at a time and then settling him in the other part of the bed where he will continue to sweat. If the procedure has been carried out well and the influenza is in its initial stage, the patient will recover full health. Of course, there must be someone who looks after him, because this is not a treatment that can be done alone.

Besides, one of the deeper spiritual meanings of illness is that of promoting mutual help among mankind.

Basic drugs for influenza

There are many useful remedies for influenza. One of the most important in the anthroposophic tradition is *Bryonia/Eucalyptus comp. drops*. These drops are a combination of the main remedies that help to tolerate the symptoms of influenza better, in particular, phosphorus, which has a specific effect of supporting the sensory system, so often affected in influenza. The dose is 10-12 drops every hour, while the fever is high; the frequency of administration is then gradually reduced to every two hours, then every three hours, until three or four times a day. It is important not to withdraw this treatment too early or indeed suspend the bed rest and light diet. It is always preferable to extend the treatment for one more day.

In children, on the other hand, it is better to use the already mentioned *Ferrum phosphoricum comp. globules*, 2-5 globules every two hours while the fever is still present, and then slowly tapering down the dose, as for the drops in adults. The globules, which do not contain alcohol, are very practical and are often also used with benefit in adults at a dose of 10-15 globules every hour. This treatment lacks the strong neurosensory support provided by pure phosphorus, since the globules only contain iron phosphate, but nevertheless, remains a good remedy.

As far as concerns controlling the patient's temperature, follow the advice given in the chapter on fever.

The convalescence
After being struck by influenza, it would be very important to have a true period of convalescence, even if brief. Unfortunately, the pace of our daily life does not allow this, which is a great pity, because the body really needs a period of recovery, which would allow an influenza to be transformed into an occasion for purification and strengthening of defences. We do at least try to let our children have a proper convalescence, not sending them to school for one or two days after the fever has disappeared, but leaving them to have an appropriate period of rest that enables full recovery of their nervous system that has been weakened by the illness.

Contagion
We all know that influenza is connected to viruses, which are transmitted from person to person in the air and through droplets of saliva.

We are, however, convinced that this plays a secondary role and that the contagion derives from a quality of our ether body, which has a natural tendency to imitate what it encounters and does so also in the case of the illnesses in which we come in contact: in fact, this is the real source of contagion, together with the weakness of the nerve-sense system, seasonal factors (cold, dampness) and cosmic factors (planetary conjunctions that decrease the protective effect of sunlight) and finally with the material presence of the virus. This makes it easy to understand why, when a child sneezes in a classroom and that sneeze, like a potent aerosol, spreads hundreds and millions of virus to every child in the room, in the following days, only some of the children will develop the influenza: viruses alone are not sufficient to produce a contagion, but they must be accompanied by a weakened nerve-sense system, which lowers the defences and the capacity to overcome viral attacks on a daily basis.

Sore throat

We have already approached this area of illness when we spoke about persistent colds, that is, when the inflammatory process, starting from the rhinopharynx, invades the true pharynx and/or the tonsils. I would like to point out that in this case we have an acute inflammatory process in the upper pole of the person: where there is inflammation, there is a change in the relationship between the person's constituent processes.

Let us take a look at the *four stages of inflammation*, which were recognized at the dawn of Hippocratic medicine, in relationship to the already described *four constituent parts of the human being*:

CALOR (warmth)	"I"
DOLOR (pain)	ASTRAL
TUMOR (swelling)	ETHER
RUBOR (redness)	PHYSICAL

The treatment of inflammation of the throat is aimed at restoring a balance between the constituent parts, taking into account the subdivision of man into three functional systems:

Upper pole: the nerve-sense system	HEAD	SAL
Unifying region: the cardiorespiratory rhythmic system	RHYTHM	MERCUR
Lower pole: the metabolic-limb system	METABOLISM	SULPHUR

In essence, with a sore throat we have a dominance, an invasion of the metabolic process into the sphere of the nerves and senses: between the upper pole and the lower pole, there is a unifying region at the level of the heart. *It is here that the equilibrium must be restored, returning the constituent parts of the person into their mutual functional spheres.*

All the inflammatory disorders of the respiratory tract, such as

Sore throat

tonsillitis, tracheitis and bronchitis, are treated in the first place with a *therapy that diverts downwards*, which works by restoring the equilibrium between the head and the abdomen. The sovereign remedy is the *purge*.

In this context, the principle of a *hot footbath*, already described for colds, should be understood as a therapy aimed at drawing the metabolic forces downwards. *Castor oil* is an excellent remedy (unless, obviously, the patient has intestinal complications) for re-balancing the metabolism in the abdominal region, which depleted of its forces no longer works well. *Laxatives should be avoided in febrile patients*.

When a fever is present, the treatment indicated, particularly in children, is an *enema*. A purge is recommended only in the case that the child suffers from an illness derived from overeating "heavy" foods such as chocolate, cured meats, chips, and industrially produced desserts and drinks, all manifested by the typical "dirty" tongue.

However, in general, an enema is a valid remedy for the initial stage of illnesses of the respiratory tract; for the doctor who has to treat such illnesses this treatment is a considerable aid because the course of the illness will be less acute since the healing forces present in the metabolism will already be mobilised.

Modern research has demonstrated that the body's most extensive defence system is in the bowel: in fact, this is the largest site of our immune system.

A sore throat is often the consequence of repeated abuse of food, which is why the frequency of tonsillitis and pharyngitis increases during the major festivities, precisely when we tend to overeat, filling ourselves with meals that are too rich and too sweet.

An enema can relieve the situation and make the clinical picture less dramatic.

Besides enemas and a correct diet, another useful remedy in the stage preceding the illness is:

Echinacea tablets. In children over two or three years old, dissolve half a tablet in the mouth, three or four times a day; older children, over six or seven years old, can be given a whole tablet three or four times a day. Extremely useful in the cold season, this is a typical anthroposophic remedy: the prevailing idea is not that of associating the activities of various plants, but to combine them to create a new product, a new therapy: in this case we are working with the composite family of flowers, of which the best known example is the common daisy. Besides *Echinacea angustifolia*, which is an immunostimulant, these tablets contain *calendula*, *chamomile* and *eucalyptus essential oil*. All this has a balsamic and refreshing effect and helps the breathing.

Enemas: instructions for use. Allow me to give some indications, since being prescribed a simple enema can cause panic in some people. I recommend using an *enema bag for bowel irrigation*, where the water descends and enters the bowel under the force of gravity, rather than an *enema bulb*, where we exert the pressure and air is inevitably introduced into the bowel together with the fluid[20].

First a tea of chamomile flowers is prepared (using a tablespoon of flowers for every half litre of water) pouring the flowers into boiling water and then leaving the liquid covered for a long time, both because the preparation should be administered lukewarm and because this accentuates the muscle-relaxing effect of the chamomile, which is only released after a long period of infusion. The liquid is then filtered and poured into the bag, after having checked the position of the stopcock. Between a quarter and three-quarters of a litre of fluid should be used. Despite our uncertainties, we must not be afraid: a child's bowel is not that small, as can be readily appreciated by the size of his faeces. The enema is administered with the patient lying down. The bag should be held high, perhaps hooked to a shower unit. The nozzle should, of course, be lubricated with a bit of olive oil to help it slip into the anus.

One piece of good advice is not to open the stopcock complete-

---

[20] A small bulb enema can be useful for young babies who need a mild stimulus to help them pass a motion.

ly, so that the liquid flows down more slowly: this will cause fewer contractions and the fluid will reach further up the bowel having a more profound effect.
For adults: use about 1.5-2 litres of tea of chamomile flowers.
I recommend administering the enema very slowly to obtain a very deep effect, approaching that of colonic irrigation which is all the rage these days.
For children: other ingredients can be added to the chamomile tea. For example, for children from two to six years old I prescribe a *pinch of bicarbonate* and a *teaspoon of sugar*, to compensate for any acidosis that is often related to the fever and rich foods eaten in the preceding days.

Medical treatment of the sore throat in children
A basic remedy for a sore throat, particularly in children who, in most cases, have tonsillitis, is a combination of two anti-inflammatory treatments such as *Apis* and *Belladonna*. This is an important background therapy to control the inflammation. A preparation containing mercury is added to act specifically on the mucosa. These two remedies are used in alternation. We can give:
Apis D3 drops;
Belladonna D4 drops;
Mercurius vivus naturalis D6 tablets.
Depending on the age of the patient, from 3 to 6 drops of each of the first two remedies (*Apis, Belladonna*) are put into a small amount of water and are given, in alternation, every two or three hours, with half a tablet of *Mercurius vivus naturalis D6* to be dissolved in the mouth; a whole tablet is used for children over 7-8 years old. If the fever is high, the treatment can be given in alternation ever hour until the temperature lowers and the inflammation resolves; at this point we can gradually prolong the interval between doses of the treatment to every two hours, then every three hours, until reaching three times a day for a few days.
There are also remedies in the form of *globules*:
Apis/Belladonna;
Apis/Belladonna cum Mercurio.

In this case the dose is from 3 to 10 globules every two or three hours, or, in the case of a high fever, every hour.

Since these remedies do not contain alcohol, they are very easy to give. The inclusion of mercury in the second remedy makes the treatment simple and complete, although administering mercury separately has a more profound and incisive effect. Both these treatments are useful for initial treatment, but if the illness is more challenging, the doctor will proceed to other more radical treatments.

I would also remind you of *Echinacea/Mercurius comp. suppositories*. These are very useful for resolving inflammation, but also for giving the immune system a stimulus. Suppositories based on natural compounds are, however, only effective when the mucosa is clean, that is, after an enema. Suppositories are used once or twice a day and given in association with the other remedies described, they enhance the effect of these latter.

The treatment for tonsillitis and other important illnesses must not be stopped abruptly, but continued into the first stage of the convalescence. For example, the *Mercurius* therapy can be continued two or three times a day for one or two weeks, even when the child has gone back to school.

Naturally the question of lifestyle is fundamental, in that we have said that a sore throat has its roots in the metabolism and its development is often facilitated by an inappropriate diet that weakens the intestinal immune system. For this reason we believe that enemas are indispensable, just as is a *semiliquid diet* almost completely lacking proteins, but based on fresh fruit juices, squeezed fruit and stewed fruit which help the young patient by providing him with vitamins and minerals without overtasking his digestion with proteins and fats. Once the child's condition has improved, he can move on to light rice dishes with a drop of oil and a little parsley (rich in vitamin C) and to lettuce, carrots or boiled chicory as vegetables. Protein-based foods, such as cheese, pulses, meat and fish should only be re-introduced when the child has fully recovered. Do not hurry, because real healing takes time, but pays off in the end.

Pharyngitis in the adult

The mercury-based preparations act on the real inflammatory process, preventing it from expanding beyond its limits.

One remedy that has been found to be effective is *Cinnabar*, which is mercury sulphide; this restores equilibrium (homeostasis) to the catarrhal secretory processes, also in sites where the circulation and respiration converge, such as in the lungs.

Cinnabar D6 tablets: in acute processes 1 tablet is used every three hours for a few days, which is basically 4-5 tablets a day, dissolved in the mouth.

Cinnabar D20 tablets: these are used in chronic processes or when, as already mentioned, an inflammation tends to persist, such as in the case of rhinitis that becomes complicated by the development of pharyngitis. The dose is 1 tablet three to four times a day.

Pyrites/Cinnabar (D2/D20) tablets: this is a combined remedy with an extensive effect from the pharynx to the larynx. It is used in cases of inflammation of the pharynx and trachea with a noisy, irritating cough. The dose is 1 tablet three to five times a day.

Causticum Hahnemanni D6 or *D30 drops*: this traditional homeopathic remedy is used in the case of a burning pain on both sides of the throat, which is often accompanied by a very persistent dry cough. Ten drops are given every two to three hours.

Generally speaking, a mercury-based therapy is usually sufficient in an adult. This treatment should be continued for one week after the acute phase has passed, reducing the frequency of administration to two or three times a day and accompanying the drops with life style measures such as a light diet, a purge, and/or enema. In the case of fever, adults too can use *Apis D3* and *Belladonna D4 drops*: 6 drops of each combined and alternated with a mercury-based preparation such as *Cinnabar D6*.

Local remedies for a sore throat

A useful remedy, unjustly neglected in favour of sprays that are more expensive and less effective, but much more convenient I am afraid, is: *Bolus Eucalypti comp. powder* (10 grams are prepared with *Apis* m.t. 0.1 g, *Belladonna* m.t. 0.02 g, *Eucalyptus* m.t. 0.1 g, *Bolus alba* 9.97 g).

This harmonious composition of various anti-inflammatory agents with white clay is an effective emollient and reduces inflammation.

Gargles and *mouth washes* are prepared using a teaspoon of the powder in a glass of warm water. The preparation is left in the bathroom, covered by a saucer, and used several times a day, taking care to stir it each time, because the powder deposits on the bottom. This is an excellent remedy for inflammation of the gums and the mucosal membranes in general.

The eucalyptus lives in light, warm environments and its absorbing power is used to reclaim swamps: we can imagine that it has a similar beneficial effect on the throat.

A spray that has a good local rebalancing effect on the tonsils, particularly when there is a white cheesy-type secretion (resembling cottage cheese), is *Echinacea comp. spray*, which should be sprayed on the tonsils two or three times a day. This is also useful in the acute phase of tonsillitis with plaques, together with the internal remedies described above.

A useful remedy for gargling is *sage tea* to which the juice of half a *squeezed lemon* is added; the tea is kept in the bathroom and gargled two or three times a day. Mouth rinses are extremely useful for inflammation of the gums.

Sage is an excellent remedy for infections of the respiratory tract, so this tea can also be drunk two or three times a day.

We have deliberately not talked about throat swabs or any blood or urine tests, which are essential in cases of suspected streptococcal tonsillitis, since these are the competence of the doctor who should be consulted for any important illness.

Subglottic laryngitis or false croup

I would like to say immediately that *supraglottic laryngitis* or *acute epiglottitis* is a rare, potentially fatal disease with an acute onset that worsens rapidly. It predominantly affects children between 3 and 6 years old. The alarm signs are stridor, the noisy inspiratory breathing that can be heard even at a distance, laboured breathing manifested by retraction of the skin in the spaces between the ribs, throat and diaphragm, fast breathing, high fever and saliva drooling from the mouth because the child cannot swallow. If these signs are present, the child should be taken immediately to an Accident and Emergency department for the appropriate treatment, such as cortisone, a drip for rehydration, oxygen and antibiotics. I list these drugs to emphasise that in these cases they are essential and should be exploited without limitation. Sometimes the signs are caused by an allergic-type swelling of the glottis, which also requires prompt admission to hospital.

In contrast, *subglottic laryngitis* or *false croup* is a common illness in children that causes alarm in parents and often also in young doctors. In this case the inflammation is below the glottis; there is stridor, but no pain on swallowing and if there is a fever, it is a low-grade one. *I advise that you call your own doctor.* In fact, this is a benign illness that can be treated and cured perfectly with anthroposophic remedies. The child wakes up before or around midnight, inspiring noisily with a characteristic stridor; when he coughs he makes a sound resembling the barking of a dog. He will often hold his throat, cry hoarsely and is very frightened. We are dealing with a child who is normally healthy, who has probably played all afternoon outside, sweated, and towards evening, when the sun has set and the temperature has dropped, begins to feel cold. The same effect can occur if a child leaves a heated room to go outside in the open air on a very cold day, for example running out from a warm classroom at nursery school into the playground. In brief, instead of the nose and lungs becoming cold, the child catches cold in the larynx. The diagnosis is also based on the frequency of the symptoms: it is unlikely that a child has a severe disease every 15 days. It is more likely that frequent illnesses are false croup. While waiting to see the doctor, you should switch on the bedroom light, get the child to sit upright in bed, covering him well, and put two or three cushions behind his back, but most of all, reassure him. It is also useful to get him to breathe in humid air, for example taking him into the bathroom where the bath is being filled with steaming water. At the same time, compresses soaked in hot water can be applied continuously to the child's larynx (throat). One way of doing this is to a soak a sponge glove, folded length-wise, in a bowl of hot water, wring it and, once tolerable, place it on the child's throat covering it with a dry towel; this procedure is repeated approximately every 10 minutes, taking care that the sponge glove does not become cold. This treatment should be continued until the cough changes from a continuous, barking, hoarse, dry cough into a less frequent, chesty (productive) cough; at this point, the child usually drops off to sleep to recover. The doctor will prescribe remedies to be given at the same time as the local treatment. In practice, the drops or granules prescribed should be given every five minutes. Typical remedies are *Spongia D6 drops* and *Spongia D3 granules*. Subsequently the same treatment is given four or five times a day for the next two or three days.

Laryngospasm is a mild form of subglottic laryngitis, often of viral origin. Children with a tendency to allergies may have recurrent episodes, particularly during the night. Your doctor should be consulted in any case.

Sinusitis

I believe that sinusitis is a neglected and under-diagnosed illness, which is why I would like to dedicate particular attention to it here.

The human head, where the nerve-sense system dominates, contains numerous hollows spaces full of air, called the *paranasal sinuses*. The nose is an "enclave", situated in the head, of the central rhythmic system of man; in fact, it communicates directly with the thorax through the airways.

All the paranasal sinuses, cavities lined by respiratory tract-like mucosa, arise as protrusions of the nasal mucosa in the embryonic period, at the same time as the appearance of the teeth. This is the start of a long process that takes place in the first three seven-year periods of life. Just consider that it is the paranasal sinuses that enlarge the face, giving it its human appearance and contributing to the definitive physiognomy of the face.

These cavities are still very small in the neonate and young baby and the frontal sinuses are completely absent.

At every stage of development of these sinuses there is a transformation in the consciousness and these organs can become diseased. The time of formation and pneumatisation (penetration of air into these cavities, or, anthroposophically, penetration of the astral body whose medium is air) of the paranasal sinuses means that the ethmoid sinuses tend to be affected early, already from the second or third year of life. This is the period in which a child's consciousness undergoes a big change when, as Steiner's knowledge of man teaches us, the child starts saying "I" to refer to himself. The maxillary sinuses can become affected from the start of the second seven-year period of life, coinciding with the child's development having reached the point of being ready to go to school.

The sphenoid sinuses are fully formed around the time of puberty, which is accompanied by an important evolution in the wakeful consciousness and sexual development. At that point the frontal sinuses also complete their formation, with the birth of the astral body whose physical medium, as we have said, is air, the gaseous element.

The completion of the development of these cavities containing free air, in the adolescent, gives the astral body the possibility to free itself from the metabolic processes, to be available for the person's sentimental life. The frontal sinus is fully developed at around the age of twenty years.

Only when the level of consciousness approaches that of an adult can there be a real attack of frontal sinusitis. All the sinuses form a single functional unit and are the base for the action of the astral body; for this reason, any change in them is accompanied by varying degrees of modification of the consciousness.

The *initial symptoms of sinusitis* are the same as the typical signs of infections of the upper airways, such as sneezing, rhinitis, dulled consciousness and a headache that varies depending on the site of the sinusitis.

Frontal sinusitis causes pain in the area of the forehead and a frontal headache.

Maxillary sinusitis causes pain in the area of the upper jaw, toothache and a frontal headache.

Ethmoid sinusitis causes pain behind and between the eyes and a violent frontal headache in the case of a restless child with a fever; a discharge of pus on the posterior wall of the rhinopharynx raises the suspicion of ethmoiditis. *In contrast, in school age, this symptom accompanied by facial pain suggests a possible maxillary sinusitis.*

A child with frequent headaches can often be helped by discovering that the underlying diagnosis is sinusitis and treating this root cause of his problem.

The pain related to *sphenoid sinusitis* is less well localised and is referred to the frontal or occipital area.

A fever and feeling cold can both be expressions of extension of the disease to other areas of the body. A high fever with a strong headache are common signs of a sinusitis that has complicated a neglected influenza.

Sinusitis

The marked tendency to recurrent sinusitis is explained by the modern-day, irrational desire to stay on one's feet at all costs, the adolescents' habit of not covering themselves up properly when it is cold, and the abuse of antibiotics, which are often needlessly self-prescribed for viral infections.

Finally, the connection between the paranasal sinuses and the astral body, the carrier of the soul life, explains why this illness is overlooked by affected patients who, every autumn, telephone full of concern and anxiety about a "mysterious" headache that has developed after a banal cold. A doctor who keeps good clinical records can help a patient to recognize an illness that his soul wants to forget. How many times have I had to show a patient that this was the third or fourth time that this mysterious illness recurred! How many times have my patients consulted therapists of every sort, from neurologists to osteopaths, receiving the most variegated set of diagnoses for an illness that we have already known about for years!

This "psychological forgetfulness" is common in patients who have a severe illness such as a tumour and, therefore, have a weak warmth body in the cranial pole.

The main cause of sinusitis is coldness of the peripheral parts of the body, particularly the upper pole: dissipation of warmth weakens the organization of "I".

The nasal mucosa swells, obstructing entry to the sinus, the oxygen imprisoned is absorbed by the blood vessels of the mucosal membranes, the negative pressure within the sinus (vacuum sinusitis) causes pain because of the force separation of the astral body from the organization of "I", the mucosa produces a transudate that floods the sinus, evicting the astral body and enabling the ether body to take over. The excess of fluid forms a culture medium for pathogenic microbes. At this point the pain derives from positive pressure in the obstructed sinus.

Treatment consists fundamentally in supplying warmth that enables the organization of "I", which is linked to the body through warmth, to regain dominance of a part of the body which had escaped its control.

External treatments

Horseradish. Horseradish has a root that causes tingling and burning with the sensation of intense warmth.

External applications, over one or more maxillary or frontal sinuses, of compresses based on freshly grated horseradish root are extraordinarily effective. The grated root is placed in the centre of a cloth kept closed with a sticking plaster: this compress brings forth an external inflammation which pulls the internal inflammatory process to the exterior, in this way freeing the excess ether forces in an inappropriate site and allowing the rhythmic system to restore a balance between opposing processes.

Beware of burns! In any case, this treatment should only be used once a day.

The first application should be left in place for only a few minutes in order to understand the strength of the root and evaluate the reaction of the patient's skin. The patient should hold the compress in place by hand, in order to be able to remove it when it starts to burn, as it inevitably will.

The fresh root is only available in autumn and at the beginning of winter, but this is precisely the period of sinusitis.

The first applications should not last longer than about ten minutes.

The patient should be aware that a red mark will remain on the brow or cheeks for a few days.

Powdered horseradish can also be used; this does not act as intensely, but also does not cause burns. I have treated cases of sinusitis recurring for thirty years, healing them completely with applications of this compress every autumn, for two or three years, at intervals of 10-15 days. One of my patient's garden is now overrun with horseradish, with its really tenacious roots, after I advised him to plant it because he had suffered from sinusitis for years. He is now very satisfied with the results obtained, and tolerates this invasive, but healing plant. *Note that this is a challenging treatment, only suitable for adults.*

Mustard. A compress made with mustard flour has the same indications as the horseradish compress and can be used to reinforce this latter's action. It is, however, better that this is prescribed by your doctor.

Flaxseed (linseed). In chronic forms of sinusitis, a hot poultice with linseed meal can be useful to dissolve stagnant secretions. The poultice, which is much gentler than the previous two compresses, should be repeated periodically. It is worth using organic linseed, rather than the ready-made linseed meal which is not very effective. The seeds can be ground in a coffee grinder or in a blender, for just a few seconds: they only need to be crushed, not pulverised to avoid producing a mash. Put a few spoons of the resulting meal in a small pan, mix with water as if to make semolina and heat, without letting the mixture boil otherwise the poultice will lose its efficacy. Put the hot poultice in the middle of a thick napkin and fold over the four sides as if making a package and then close it with a sticking plaster. Apply the poultice to the forehead, first with the side more protected by the folds on the skin and then with the other, less protected side. Place a towel over the poultice package in order to keep the warmth in.

For the maxillary sinuses, close two balls of the poultice, about as big as table-tennis balls, into the napkin and then apply them to the face over the cheekbones. Hold them there for at least 15-20 minutes.

Inhalations/hot vapour treatments. Hot, humid vapours prepared with bicarbonate together with an tea of chamomile are useful to relieve pain. Prepare a generous amount of a strong tea of chamomile and, after having filtered it, add a spoonful of bicarbonate. Hold the head over a large cup or pan containing the tea and cover the head with a towel to keep in the heat and humidity. *When using this treatment for children, you should wait until the inhalation has cooled slightly,* and in any case, great care should be taken that the child is not scalded as a result of abrupt movements. Obviously the adult must also go under the towel, holding the child in his arms; this treatment must be made into a tent game of "playing Indians", not a restraint.

Inhalations of essential oils of lemon or eucalyptus, which have disinfectant and astringent effects on swollen mucosal membranes, are always interesting. Always use a few drops diluted in physiological saline, because essential oils are effective but very irritant.

As already mentioned, horseradish or mustard compresses are always useful for pain.

Carex arenaria 1% ointment. This ointment is valuable for "drawing out" an inflammation and also has a soothing effect.

It can be used for long-term treatment, applying it on the forehead and over the cheekbones in the evenings.

Medical treatment

Anthroposophic doctors agree in indicating *Argentum/Berberis comp. ampoules* as a fundamental remedy for sinusitis. This compound actually combines three essential remedies: *berberis*, a remedy that is typically targeted at the astral body, with its connection with the rhinopharyngeal region and the kidneys-bladder, *silver*, a great regulator of inflammation, and finally, *quartz*, to contain and support the formative process modified by the inflammation. This remedy is very effective, but must be prescribed by your doctor who, sometimes, should give the first local injections personally.

In the case of tenacious secretions, I recommend *Kalium bichromicum D6 drops*, 10 drops four or five times a day. Another very useful remedy is the homeopathic preparation *Nuspax*: one tablet every two or three hours, to chew or dissolve in the mouth: this promotes secretion and soothes pain.

For children, but also for adults with milder forms of sinusitis, a first-choice treatment while waiting to see the doctor is:

Berberis/Quartz granules, 5 granules (10 for adults) to be taken every two hours, reducing the dose after two or three days to once every three or four hours and possibly alternating this with a tablet of *Nuspax* in the more relevant cases.

Aloe (Rhinodoron) nasal spray. This is very useful for moisturising and cleaning the nasal passages; the aloe gel helps to regenerate the nasal mucosae. This spray can also be used for babies who are unable to blow their nose.

For the delicate skin of children, *linseed meal poultices* can be applied locally to the area involved, followed by or alternated with applications of *Carex arenaria 1%* ointment.

Prevention
It is essential that the hands and feet of children are kept protected from the cold. Warm footbaths are always useful, for adults as well. Powdered ginger, for example, can be added to the footbaths.
One simple, but useful piece of advice for all patients who have had an episode of sinusitis, but even more so for those who tend to have recurrent attacks or a chronic form of the illness, is to wear a hat (which doesn't necessarily have to cover the forehead) throughout the cold season, because this reduces the efforts that the warmth body has to expend in warming the head.
Finally, a treatment that acts on the liver, the great regulator of the fluid component of the body, is often very beneficial in preventing recurrences. However, your doctor is needed for such treatment.
It is important to help your doctor, both by keeping wrapped up well and by following a healthy diet, so that in the autumn and, in particular, during the winter, you eat foods that support your body by supplying warmth rather than by dissipating it. In this sense, the *Solanaceae* (peppers, aubergines and tomatoes), eaten during the cold season, weaken the warmth body, while the *cruciferous* vegetables (radish, broccoli, pumpkin, cabbage, cauliflower, celery, turnip, etc.) have the opposite effect of reinforcing the processes retaining warmth in the body. In recent years these vegetables have gained great prestige in the medical world, given the pronounced support of the immune system that they offer those who eat them. They are also considered the vegetables that have the greatest protective effects against tumours.

The cough: an unwelcome defence mechanism

The cough: the tip of the iceberg of an illness
I do not want to dedicate too much space to this subject, which is a really thorny issue in the relationship, particularly over the telephone, between doctors and patients: I cannot think of anything as omnipresent in my daily clinical activity as the unremitting requests to make a cough disappear. Whether we are talking about adults or children, it seems that our society poorly tolerates this symptom, often leading us to accept any proffered treatment, from sorcery to codeine syrup, which is a drug, in order to free ourselves of this "visible sound" and make us well and silent at work just as in public gardens. The contradiction lies in the fact that a cough is tolerated by very few people, but is seldom considered a symptom sufficient to take to the doctor. This, sometimes, leads to late diagnoses, which necessitate aggressive treatments of limited effectiveness, such as the prescription of antibiotics. Such treatments are inappropriate when, as is often the case, the cough is caused by a virus or the cough continues after the bacterial infection has already been overcome.
Cough is undoubtedly one of the most common symptoms and can be related to numerous illnesses of the upper and lower respiratory tracts. The first important point to make is that a cough is essentially a defence mechanism, shared by many cardiorespiratory disorders, aimed at eliminating secretions and foreign bodies from the trachea and bronchi. It is caused by a mechanical or chemical stimulus of a very large reflex-generating area (pharynx, larynx, trachea, main bronchi). The act of coughing has several phases: a deep inspiration, closure of the glottis, contraction of muscles and an expulsive expiration. During the act of coughing, the pressure within the thorax increases greatly and, in the long term, this can have repercussions, sometimes serious, on the circulatory system. A cough accompanied by the expulsion of catarrh during a bronchopulmonary infection or inflammation should not be suppressed, but rather, it should be promoted with

remedies with an expectorant effect (encouraging expectoration) in order to free the airways. In contrast, a dry, irritating cough, particularly in a patient with a heart condition, should be promptly suppressed with appropriate medicaments. A dry cough that persists in the absence of other symptoms may be a sign of a mediastinal syndrome and require careful medical assessment. It will be the task of the doctor, by analysing the characteristics of the cough and any other symptoms that may be present (fever, difficulty in breathing, presence of secretions, phlegm), to diagnose the underlying disease; the most common causes of an acute cough include the cold-related illnesses, acute pharyngitis, acute tracheitis, acute bronchitis and allergic diseases. If, however, the cough has been present for a long time (chronic cough), is resistant to symptomatic treatments and is accompanied by a general malaise, it is worth carrying out some diagnostic investigations, including chest X-rays. We anthroposophic doctors, who use analyses and investigations with moderation, often have to insist to make it understood that in this case the diagnosis must be clarified; for example, viral pneumonias cannot be picked up by auscultation and can only be diagnosed by X-rays. The causes of a chronic cough obviously include pneumonia, chronic bronchitis, allergies, bronchiectasis, granulomatous diseases and malignancies.

The cough and home remedies
An acute cough is mainly related to infections of the upper and lower respiratory tracts. First of all, the underlying illness can be treated using familiar home remedies (refer to the chapters on colds, influenza and sore throat); once the underlying illness has been resolved, the cough becomes less important to the body and tends to disappear *slowly*. We must be patient, because excessive treatment can often have the paradoxical effect of hampering recovery and actually making the cough necessary. I sometimes remain astonished by the therapeutic arsenal unleashed against an innocent cough that, at the end of a bout of pharyngitis or influenza, is helping the body to clean up. Sometimes, with con-

trasting actions we swing the balance of the mucosa too far towards the liquid: then the cough will reappear to accelerate the removal of the excessive secretions produced. In contrast, the use of expectorants when the mucous membranes are drying up will cause a chesty, wet cough, so we are starting all over again. Various preparations for treating a cold also contain a cough inhibitor, which, while there might be sense in prescribing to a person with heart disease, becomes counterproductive in a child. Let's consider this question: why do we want to interfere with a natural mechanism for expelling the catarrh that is congesting a child's lungs? We have said that a cough, which occurs in all the diseases of the airways, is a defence mechanism to eliminate excessive mucus and inhaled foreign matter (powders, germs, pollen, etc.). There are some areas of the airways (larynx, trachea) that are more sensitive than others to foreign substances of any type; even minimal stimulation of these areas provokes intense coughing, particularly a dry cough. A separate situation occurs in small babies who, unable to cough efficiently, have great difficulty in expelling phlegm. The cough often disturbs the baby, even when sleeping, and sometimes causes vomiting.

In the presence of catarrh, the cough, which in this case is called *chesty, wet* or *productive*, serves to remove mucous and microbes from the airways and is, therefore, a defence mechanism that should be maintained. When there are no secretions and the cough derives from irritation of the more sensitive parts of the airways (throat, larynx and trachea), it is called a *dry* cough.

The *first measure* to relieve this discomfort is to maintain a *high level of humidity in the room* and, indeed, throughout the house. A humidifier can be useful for this purpose, provided that it is clean, otherwise it will release an irritant mist. A few drops of vinegar are added to the specific container to prevent the growth and spread of fungi. If the child has difficulty in breathing through his nose, or if he has a barking cough, take him into the bathroom, close the door, open the shower fully and make the child breathe the steam for twenty minutes.

We must also take care to replace the liquids that the child loses

The cough: an unwelcome defence mechanism

when coughing, sneezing and sweating. We must make him drink a good glass of liquid every hour: fruit juices, or better still fresh fruit whisked together with water and honey, are excellent for restoring mineral salts that have been lost.

An excellent drink is *Buckthorn syrup*, which is very rich in natural vitamin C and is also mildly expectorant; we recommend one or two tablespoons diluted in a glass of water.

We can give *Blackthorn syrup* when we want to revive a child who has been particularly drained by the illness, as occurs, for example, in whooping cough; in this case, a *Fir balsam bath* can also be taken to give vitality to the skin, another organ that is important in respiration.

We must remember that a patient with a cough, whether adult or child, must drink sufficiently. In fact, most of the effects that are obtained with medicines can be achieved by working on the degree of hydration of the patient on the one hand and the humidity of the environment on the other hand.

Besides fresh fruit juices, another excellent remedy is a *lime blossom tea* (see the chapter on colds and cold-related illnesses), to which honey and freshly squeezed lemon juice can be added. This pleasant combination, which meets the needs of the feverish child, is made by adding the honey when the infusion is lukewarm and ready to be sipped by the child. I shall never tire of repeating that these drinks must be warm: cold drinks and food must be avoided because they irritate the stomach, particularly if it is empty.

Coltsfoot leaves (*Tussilago farfara* L.). A tea of this plant, whose botanical name derives from the Latin *tussis agere*, that is "drive out the cough", not only has an anti-inflammatory effect, but also thins bronchial catarrh. It has the distinction of also being effective in spasmodic forms of coughing and, therefore, in cases of whooping cough and spasmodic bronchitis. A tablespoonful of coltsfoot leaves is placed in a quarter of a litre of boiling water and left to infuse for ten minutes, covering the liquid with a lid to keep it hot in order that the leaves can release their precious mucilage. The recommended dose for adults is one cupful three to five times a day, while that for children is half a cup of the tea, which can be sweetened with honey while warm.

Thyme (Thymus vulgaris L.), flowering plant. Galen had already attributed this plant with expectorant properties; it can be used as the only ingredient in a tea, but also combines well with coltsfoot leaves, thus having a bacteriostatic effect that combats the proliferation of bacteria. There are numerous studies demonstrating the antibacterial activity of essential oils of aromas and medicinal plants[21]. A thyme tea is useful in most cases of bronchitis, which are almost always caused by viruses, and in the respiratory complications of influenza, which is also a viral infection. A tablespoonful of the flowering plant is poured into a quarter of a litre of boiling water and left to infuse for ten minutes. To make the combined thyme and coltsfoot tea, use one teaspoonful of thyme and one of coltsfoot. The dose is a cupful of tea from three to five times a day.

Coughs with insufficient expectorate (dry coughs)

Besides the teas described above, in the case of a dry cough we can use:

Bryonia D3 drops. This plant, which has a large root with small flowers and leaves, is the source of a sovereign remedy for controlling the development of fluids in inappropriate places, which is precisely what occurs in inflammation of the respiratory tract, since fluids replace air. These drops help to mature the cough and are, therefore, indicated above all in the initial phase when there

---

[21] Some laboratories now perform an *aromatogram* to determine which essential oil is most indicated for the illness affecting the patient; this investigation is widely used in recurrent bladder infections in which the use of numerous antibiotics leads, in the long run, to the selection of microbes resistant to many antibiotics, as shown by an antibiogram. The first essential oil that was used as a bacteriostatic was lemon essential oil which, in contact with bacterial cultures, showed a strong capacity to block the reproduction of the bacteria; these experiments laid the basis for the production of the famous disinfectant, *Citrosil,* in the 1930s. The antiviral effect of thyme essential oil and melissa oil are well-known. These oils are also effective when applied locally in the case of *Herpes virus* and are also used in traditional medicine.

is a dry, wracking cough which may even cause chest pain or a headache. The dose is 10 drops every two or three hours. This is also an important remedy in children, in whom the dose is obvious decreased: 3-5-7 drops every two or three hours.

Kalium bichromicum D6 drops. These are used for a cough that involves the upper part of the throat, with a stringy, viscous, yellow or green secretion coming from the nose and the back of the pharynx. These drops are a particularly effective remedy in the case of sinusitis. *Honeyed syrup with lichens.* A teaspoon of syrup can be diluted in half a cup of hot water, creating a pleasant drink to sip every two or three hours, or the syrup can be left to dissolve directly in the mouth. This remedy is suitable for children, given its delicate, sweet flavour due to the honey and its taste of anise. It is taken at the same time as treatment in the form of drops, which may be *Bryonia* or *Kalium bichromicum*. The honeyed syrup contains a mixture of various lichens which, together with marsh mallow, are the major vegetal cough expectorants.

Icelandic lichen and marsh mallow are very effective in a tea, but I only prescribe them to adults because they are bitter and not many of today's children are prepared for such a taste. For this reason, I recommend the honeyed syrup, which is pleasant.

Irritant and spasmodic coughs

Ipecacuanha comp. drops. I would like to mention this remedy, which we can consider a broad-spectrum treatment in the sense that it is a basic remedy for whooping cough, but also has a good effect whenever there is spasmodic component to a cough, a tendency to vomiting and a "nervous" component, for example in subjects in whom the cough expresses a state of inner irritation. The dose is 5-10 drops every two or three hours for irritant bronchitis and persistent bouts of coughing. The dose is reduced in children: 3-5 drops every two or three hours.

Oleum aethereum Eucalypti comp. oil, for external use. This can be an auxiliary treatment for spasmodic coughs, but is a general remedy for inflammation of the upper airways, bronchitis and tracheitis. The oil should be applied several times onto the chest and back, massaging for a long time until it has been completely absorbed. Do not exaggerate with the dose: it is better to increase the applications during the course of the day. It is particularly useful before going to sleep, which it facilitates.

Coughs with abundant expectorate (productive or chesty)

Tartarus stibiatus D5 drops. Antimony and potassium tartrate, a remedy drawn from traditional alchemy, helps the reorganization of protein processes. *Tartarus stibiatus*, a medicament that is the complete opposite of *Bryonia*, which is given in the initial stage of an illness, is used for productive coughs with abundant expectorate that makes breathing difficult. Ten drops are administered every two or three hours; the dose is reduced to 3-5-7 drops in children, in whom the remedy plays a very important role in regulating the respiratory rhythm. It is an excellent remedy at the end of a catarrhal illness or during chronic bronchitis.

Ivy and plantain syrup. I am not a great fan of syrups, but the mixture of ivy and ribwort plantain, a plant with a great tradition in the treatment of asthma and bronchitis, has convinced me to prescribe this syrup both because of its pleasant taste and because it is appropriate in the catarrhal stage of a cough. Take one teaspoon every two to three hours with the chosen remedy in drop form.

Diet and cough

Another constant theme of treating illnesses is that of food. A sick child usually wisely refuses solid food as a sort of self-care. Let's respect his choice! How many coughs are fuelled by ultra-permissive parents who become authoritarian only when it comes to compelling a sick child to eat a lumberjack's diet[22] to which, believe me, the child is often intolerant: this creates a new cough which arises precisely from the need to eliminate excess proteins

---

[22] The Canadian lumberjack's diet is part of the history of nutrition because of its high calorie count and remains synonymous with a hypercaloric diet among us nutritionists.

The cough: an unwelcome defence mechanism

that the body cannot eliminate. We have already discussed this, when speaking about nutrition.

If a child is hungry, let's give him light food, such as a vegetable puree or semolina cooked in the blended vegetables or in water; in winter we can add oatmeal, boiling it in the puree so that it releases its precious mucilage. Milk and protein food stuffs, even worse meat, are not recommended because they use too much of the body's energy to be assimilated, taking away forces from the healing process.

Tracheobronchitis

Acute tracheobronchitis is one of the most common diseases of the respiratory tract in humans. It is an infection of the airways characterized by a cough with or without phlegm. I should mention that an acute cough is defined as one lasting less than three weeks, to distinguish it from a chronic or persistent cough. Thus a cough persisting for up to twenty days is still considered acute. In adults, in 70% of cases a cough is caused by acute infections of the upper airways, in 5% of cases by asthma and in about 6% of cases by pneumonia.

It is very important to distinguish between these three diseases and so a doctor must be consulted. Some patients with a cough may be affected by a previously undiagnosed asthma, but it is difficult to make this diagnosis in the first three weeks because patients with acute bronchitis have a non-specific, transient, hyper-reactivity of the bronchi which mimics asthma. Since pneumonia is the third cause of an acute onset cough, and potentially the most dangerous, the doctor's main aim should be to exclude the presence of pneumonia.

Acute bronchitis is an extremely common illness and occupies one of the first places with regards to outpatient work.

The illness is most frequent among children from 0 to 4 years old and in the over 65-year olds.

Since the 1980s there has been a notable increase in the incidence of asthma because of the environmental factors described in the chapter on allergies.

Part II. Illnesses and remedies

From an anatomical point of view, acute bronchitis is characterized by an acute inflammation limited to the mucosa of the trachea and bronchi. It is a typical complication of the infections following bouts of influenza and the common cold-related diseases. The upper airway is the main site of the earliest manifestations of acute bronchitis. This part of the respiratory tree acts as a filter, preventing the development of more severe infections, such as pneumonia, of the lower respiratory tract.

While waiting to see the doctor and in patients with recurrent episodes, which we can recognize because they have already been diagnosed in the past, we can use some basic remedies to prevent the illness from worsening.

Pyrites tablets;
Pyrites D3/Cinnabar D20 tablets.

These are both treatments for an inflammation of the upper airways that tends to extend downwards, such as *pharyngitis*, sore throat, but also *laryngitis* with its hoarse voice and *tracheitis* with its harsh, barking cough.

The first of these two remedies is derived from *pyrite*, an iron sulphide mineral, which is important for the sphere of breathing. In anthroposophic medicine the trachea and bronchi are connected to the planetary forces of Mars, the planet which is expressed in the metal iron; still today, the term *martial therapy* is used in mainstream medicine in many countries to indicate the administration of iron.

Iron, the metal of Mars, has a complex energy metabolism in the human body, such that one can talk of an *iron process*. The iron in this remedy stimulates the circulation, while the sulphur enters between the circulation and respiration, supporting the excretory activity that is diminished by the inflammation which slows mucociliary flow to the exterior: putting things simply, it helps the expectoration of phlegm. From an anatomical point of view, *Pyrites* is the remedy for tracheobronchitis and bronchitis.

The second remedy, consisting of pyrite and cinnabar, an ore of mercury sulphide, is able to restore an equilibrium to processes of phlegm secretion and acts, in particular, where the circulation and respiration converge, such as in the respiratory tree. Anatomically its effect is manifested at a higher level, in the pharynx and trachea: it is, therefore, a remedy suitable for colds and sore throats that tend to extend downwards and to become chronic. The dose is one tablet dissolved in the mouth two to six times a day; the dose for children is half a tablet two or three times a day. For babies, the tablets can be dissolved in a small amount of water and given by spoon every hour.

Anise-Pyrites tablets. These tablets are a remedy for inflammations such as *laryngitis* with hoarseness, *tracheitis* and *bronchitis*. The tablets consist of pyrites and toasted aniseed. Dissolve one tablet in the mouth every two or three hours. This remedy protects the bronchial mucosa, performing the useful, albeit inconspicuous task of avoiding complications. For this reason, although it is a good remedy, it is poorly understood by patients who are particularly keen on medicines that act on symptoms.

Bronchitis and febrile pneumonia

These are diseases that must be treated by a doctor, so here we give only a brief description of the initial therapeutic measures.

In the more severe cases of bronchitis with fever, while waiting to see a doctor, a good remedy to take to stimulate sweating and lower the temperature is a *tea of lime blossom and black elder,* already described in the chapters on fever and colds.

A specific herb tea for acute bronchitis is:

coltsfoot leaves, 20 g;

fennel seeds, 10 g;

flowering thyme, 20 g.

Pour two tablespoons of the mixture into half a litre of boiling water, cover and leave to rest for ten minutes, filter and sweeten with honey. The tea should be drunk warm in three or four portions during the course of the day; half-doses are recommended for children. If the bronchitis is associated with a fever, add a teaspoon of lime blossom and black elder flower to the mixture described above, in order to have a single tea containing all the ingredients. My advice is to keep the few herbs recommended in

different jars, so that the mixture can be made up as needed.
If the fever is high or a diagnosis has been made by a doctor, the *basic treatment* can be started. This treatment consists of:
Aconitum/Bryonia drops and:
Phosphorus D5 drops, together with:
Tartarus stibiatus D5 drops.
Every hour, the following remedies are administered, in alternation, in a small amount of water:
– 10 drops of *Aconitum/Bryonia*;
– a mixture of 5 drops of *Phosphorus* and 5 drops of *Tartarus stibiatus*.
The doses are reduced to 3, 5, or 7 drops in children, depending on their age.
I advise care in young children and even more so in nursing babies, because the drops contain alcohol; furthermore the level of dilution of *Aconitum*, *Bryonia* and *Phosphorus* can be too low for some children, giving rise to restlessness and anxiety. In these cases your anthroposophic doctor could prescribe higher dilutions. While waiting you could give the remedy for influenza: *Ferrum phosphoricum comp. globules*, 1 to 3 globules to be dissolved in the mouth or in water for neonates.
This is a real basic treatment for bronchitis, lacking only the iron process, which can initially be supported by *Pyrites*. The medical prescription must be followed precisely, taking care not to stop the treatment abruptly, but gradually tapering the dose down to avoid a flare up of a disease process not yet completely resolved, since relapses of bronchitis are difficult to treat.

Lemon compresses

Anthroposophic medicine makes extensive use of external treatments, which are particularly effective. Here I would like to mention lemon compresses, which are easy to prepare and are used for spasmodic bronchitis and asthma. Although we might not reach the finesse that anthroposophic nurses[23] are capable of, the

---

[23] See: Bentheim v. - Bos - Visser - de la Houssaye, *Caring for the Sick at*

remedy is prepared in the following way: lay out a terry towel on the bed and, on top of this, place a thin cotton cloth, as wide as the circumference of the patient's chest, which has been soaked in warm water with lemon juice and then wrung. The patient lies down on the cotton cloth and then the terry towel is closed around his chest. This pleasant compress can be kept in place for hours to relax the bronchial spasms. It is excellent for children.

Plantago lanceolata (ribwort plantain) ointment
This is a useful remedy for any inflammation of the bronchi and trachea: it should be rubbed on the chest several times a day and can be applied alone or after a lemon compress.

Home, SteinerBooks, Inc, New York, which describes the various external treatments used in anthroposophic medicine in great detail.

The prevention and treatment of allergies

The picture of allergies
In the last twenty to thirty years allergic illnesses have increased exponentially, such that at least one in five people are now affected by an allergy. We are all asking ourselves the reason for this increase.

Economic well-being has a price that we pay physically: consider the clear parallel between increased consumerism and the development of dental caries. Modern man reacts ever more often with allergic manifestations to the difficulty of dealing with the increasingly numerous artificial substances present in the environment or introduced into the body with food.

Allergies are spreading for a variety of reasons, which can be summarised as follows:
– an increase in environmental pollution because of the presence of harmful substances in the air and water;
– use of chemical and sometimes toxic substances in agriculture;
– massive consumption of preserved and industrially manipulated food;
– a steady increase in the use of synthetic drugs and the indiscriminate tendency to self-prescription[24];
– an increase in the excitatory aspects characteristic of modern life, which create stress and tire the human nerve-sense system[25], promoting the widespread development of irritability, restlessness, insecurity, anxiety and fears.

This causes an inner state of "alertness" which makes us react in

---

[24] In this way tons of antibiotics are produced every day and distributed between humans and animals, reaching nature and worsening the fundamental relationship between human health and bacterial flora; in fact, to be healthy, humans must have a balanced, appropriate bacterial flora within their bodies. The voluntary or involuntary consumption of antibiotics, through eating antibiotic-treated animals or from the diffusion of antibiotics in nature, alters the human intestinal bacterial flora, which is essential for life.

[25] The nervous system and the sensory organs: see the chapter 'The functional threefoldness of humans' in part I of the book.

The prevention and treatment of allergies

an exaggerated way to innocuous stimuli and underlies the typical difficulty that the allergic state has in distinguishing in a balanced way between the inner human world and the external non-human one. We need to identify what is part of our world and what is not part of it.

There are three fundamental entrances to the body: *digestion, respiration* and *sensory perception*.

Everything that penetrates our body must be radically altered in order that it does not remain alien to our inner world, but can be completely assimilated or, as we anthroposophists say, "individually humanised".

The human metabolism encapsulates the mystery of the destruction and creation of substance within man, a concept difficult to understand in the contemporary materialistic view.

Knowledge of this mystery can help us to understand the tragic errors based on the mechanistic attitudes of our times, such as feeding chickens with machinery oil or giving cows fodder made of other animals. Steiner unequivocally predicted the "mad cow" syndrome, 76 years before its appearance[26].

The phenomenon of "individual humanisation" of food is very clear in the *digestion*: everything that enters the body must, sooner or later, be completely transformed. This transformation is necessary, indeed indispensable, in order that what is ingested can be used to the benefit of the body.

What was first external becomes something that can be assimilated as a result of the process of digestion.

In order to be in balance, the body must be able to establish its control over every substance with which it comes in contact.

Our *immune system,* which controls the defence of the body, works continuously without us being aware of its existence. However, in order for the body to work well, we must reckon with our immune system, which we only notice when we fall ill. The immune system is active from birth. All the time we are unconsciously perceiving and digesting and, without realising it, we

---

[26] See: S.M. Francardo, *I semi del futuro*, Edilibri, Milano 2001, p. 41.

are becoming immune to many substances, just as we continuously transform the substances that reach us in our tissues. Both functions, perception and digestion, can exceed their normal undetected activity, giving rise to the symptoms of the illness, which can be transient or chronic.

Allergy as an illness
An *excessive activity* of the immune defence system is an indicator of processes that we call *allergic*.
If, in contrast, it is the digestive immunological process that is overstimulated, i.e., the non-specific defence (non-specific immunity) is excessive, we develop *inflammation*. We can clarify this with an example.
Hay fever is certainly one of the most widely spread allergic disorders. This disorder is a hypersensitivity to the proteins of pollen, usually from grasses, but also from trees and shrubs. In fact, hay fever is a typically seasonal allergy, occurring during the pollen season.
A baby does not have hay fever in the first year of life: at least two seasons are needed before this allergy can develop. Why? In all people, flower pollen enters the body through the mucosal membranes of the nose, throat and eyes. In these boundary zones the body, healthy or not, produces antibodies in reaction to the pollen; these antibodies serve to capture the pollen.
In the following years, an allergic person will produce excessive amounts of these antibodies.
It is interesting to note that in allergies, the production of antibodies – which in itself is a positive event, since it is a part of our defence system – becomes a source of illness if it exceeds the body's needs: illness is always an expression of an imbalance, whether this is due to a deficiency or to an excess.
An excess of antibodies leads to the development of inflammation, the purpose of which is to digest the excess antibodies produced. The allergic patient complains of burning or itching of the mucosa or skin affected. The inflammatory stimulus increases secretions, leading to the onset of colds, tears, sneezing and cough.

The prevention and treatment of allergies

Allergies start at the *periphery* of the body: for example, in the case of hay fever the allergy is manifested in the mucosal membranes of the head, while in the case of urticaria or the various forms of allergic eczema, such as atopic eczema or constitutional eczema, the symptoms start in the skin. If the disorder worsens or is blocked too abruptly by treatments which prevent the body from learning to control its boundaries with the external world, the illness extends to the *inside of the body*.

Hay fever or eczema that penetrates into the body, can appear in the form, for example, of *allergic asthma,* which is definitely a more severe form of the illness.

An allergic person has a state of what can be called hypersensitivity of the person's immune perceptive system. The perceptive activity leads to an excessive response, that is, an exaggerated production of antibodies, with the obvious consequence of overabundant formation of antigen-antibody immune complexes which accumulate in the tissues such as the mucosal membranes of the nose and throat.

In order to be able to digest this accumulation, the internal metabolism must be intensified. We therefore have the development of local inflammation, which on the level of substance, is the expression of excessive local digestive processes, manifested by the typical symptoms from redness to itching and increased secretions. It should be emphasized that the initial problem is an excessive immunological perception, but that the whole immunological system then becomes involved.

The process goes from a pathological perception to a pathological digestion. Thus, a hypersensitive perception corresponds to an illness of the nerve-sense system. The allergic person also has a notoriously hypersensitive consciousness, with regards to his soul experience[27] as such. This becomes clear if we consider that

---

[27] We prefer to use the term *soul* rather than the more commonly used *mind* because it seems to us to refer to a much broader concept than the single activity of intellectual thought which the term mind usually refers to: in fact, we refuse a conception that limits the consciousness and profound reality of man to the brain alone.

immunological perception is nothing other than the vanguard of the nerve-sense system within the metabolic pole, the system through which we gain awareness of our soul experiences. If it were only for our metabolism, we could act (muscle activity), but we could not perceive or think (sensory and nervous activities).

Prevention of allergies

As we have already said, modern day man must defend himself against numerous substances present everywhere, but in particular in food. The proliferation of irritant stimuli and the continual need to defend oneself can lead to excessive sensitivity, to reactive allergies.

It should, therefore, be understood that an allergy is based on a correct action of the body, that is, defending the body against external factors, but which occurs in an excessive, exaggerated and counterproductive way. Thus, when treating an allergy we must not try to repress this action, as is the current tendency with anti-histamines, or even worse, corticosteroids, which suppress the immune response. The truly curative solution is to try to restore a state of balance in the body: otherwise we run the risks of making the body too weak and promoting the action of the alien elements, whether they be germs or uncontrolled external stimuli: in the long term this will lead to the development of degenerative diseases such as tumours and atherosclerotic disorders.

The *diet* plays a significant role in allergies. In our industrialised era food is full of extraneous substances, lacking a proper relationship with nature: sick plants are grown, kept alive and distorted by chemical fertilisers and toxic pesticides.

A consequence of the paucity of vitality in modern foodstuffs is a progressive weakening of the human body's defences, which favours the pathogenic effect of the alien and toxic substances.

Finally, there is the problem of the *additives* used in the food industry: preservatives, antioxidants, flavour enhancers, colourants, flavourings, thickeners and gelling agents used as binders, stabilisers such as phosphates, emulsifiers, acidifiers and raising agents. These can cause *sensitisation* and *allergies*.

The tendency to react disproportionately to environmental influences often has a hereditary origin; thus, the increasing potential of modern life to cause allergies can give rise to phenomena of clustering, which worsen over time, involving whole families. In these cases (*allergic families*) it is extremely important to be prudent with irritant substances and essential to choose suitable foods in the early stages of life.

In reality, in the case of *constitutional* or *atopic eczema*, *allergic asthma* and *hay fever,* we can reasonably speak of a single illness that is manifested in different ways.

In a so-called atopic child, who can be identified based on the family history and almost always by the presence of antibodies (the levels of immunoglobulin E are high from birth), the symptoms often develop early, within the first few months of life, and it is, therefore, important to intervene right from the start.

Breastfeeding

The *primary prevention* is maternal breastfeeding, which should be defended at all costs.

We can support a mother's lactation with two calcium-based preparation:

Apatit D6 comp., consisting of a mineral, apatite, a calcium fluorophosphate and the flowers of *Cucurbita pepo*, a pumpkin. Half a coffee-spoon of the mixture, to be dissolved in the mouth, is given in the morning.

Conchae 5% comp.: this is made of *Calcium carbonicum ostrearum*, calcium carbonate derived from oyster shells, and *Quercus*, a decoction of oak bark. The dose is half a teaspoon of the mixture, to dissolve in the mouth, and should be taken in the evening.

These preparations avoid decalcification in the mother, support the production of her milk and help the baby reach an equilibrium. Calcium is a regulator of the process of mineralisation, which means that these preparations also accompany and regulate the synthesis of proteins.

Both preparations are excellent remedies for what, in children, was once called *"exudative diathesis"*, that is, the tendency to produce lymph and allergies, which was less common in the past than it is now. These remedies are therapeutically active in the two main types of allergic children, that is, lean, excitable children and stolid, sluggish ones.

Species Carvi comp., or a *tisane of cumin*, is wonderful. Although the formula of this preparation is well-known and easily copied, in clinical experience I have found that it is worth using the herbs of the original preparation, derived from well-established biodynamic agriculture. It is a *lactagogue* tisane that has the dual action of stimulating and supporting the production of milk in the mother and of making the milk more easily digested and assimilated by the baby. I advise the caring husband to take a thermos flask of this tisane to hospital so that the new mother can drink it immediately after delivery to stimulate the production of milk and to replace fluids and mineral salts. This tisane creates an elemental harmony that resonates within the mother, reaching the ether body which is in communion with that of the baby.

One of the most fascinating processes that I have encountered in my profession is precisely that of the exchange of etheric forces between mother and child, which enables us to act on the child through the mother's body. By prescribing a tisane to a mother, I can nurture the metabolism of her breastfed child.

A worthy "wait": a gift from the Gods
It is a good thing if a mother eats biodynamic food during her pregnancy, but above all that she waits in a balanced manner for her baby to be born. In this way the pregnancy can be appreciated as a gift: surrendering a small part of one's own microcosm in order that another being can create his own. Isn't giving a little bit of one's own heaven a gift of the Gods? One sign of this gift of the inner cosmos is a *decrease in the iron in a mother's blood*, which should not be considered as an illness, but as a profoundly feminine "gesture". The choice of the maternal body to decrease its iron content has a very precise meaning: that of reducing the forces of its own immune system and conscious life in or-

der to welcome, to leave a place within itself for another.

A perfect image of pregnancy can be found in the ecstatic, dreaming expressions of Raphael's portraits of the Madonna, paintings that we anthroposophic doctors recommend to expecting mothers. Enriching the dialogue with an unborn child is such a profound communion that I have no words to describe its greatness. I am, however, certain that it means giving joy to a baby and joy, as we all know, is the greatest regulator of the immune system.

In order to be superactive, a mother engages in a battle which leads her to contend for her foetus' space; such "Amazons", full of iron and strong muscles, give birth to hyperstimulated babies, babies with an immune system that feels threatened by the power of the maternal body and, therefore, produces antibodies against every manifestation of life, against every protein with which it comes into contact: this is precisely the profile of the allergic state that is sometimes found in children of women who have been efficient and active during pregnancy.

I hope it is clear that I do not intend criticising anyone – there are millions of women *forced* by work and modern social relations to be very active during their pregnancies – I just want to give voice to a point of view that has little space in modern communication. I simply ask that a woman who has the possibility to choose is not influenced by the one-track thinking that transforms a pregnancy from an event into a medical protocol. I am sure that no dialogue is established with an unborn child by watching the videocassette recording of an ultrasound.

Dietary choices and the care of allergies

By strengthening and modulating the conscious perception of the external world that enters us through food, correct dietary choices can have the effect of regulating and controlling the protective action of the immune system, which responds in an exaggerated manner in allergies. A correct diet could help to restore a balance to the immune system, without weakening it as treatment with corticosteroids and antibiotics do, since these drugs are specifically intended to inhibit or replace the work of the immune system.

For example, anthroposophic medicine teaches that a diet based on raw vegetables, and in particular on *roots*, activates a structuring force that has curative effects on skin altered by an allergy. The vegetables must, of course, be healthy, otherwise we could actually worsen the allergy by introducing into the body chemical substances used to treat the plants, in particular because such substances concentrate precisely in the roots.

A basic dietary therapy in the case of allergic reactions consists in following a wholemeal diet, that is, a diet based on biodynamic wholemeal cereals. Biodynamic wholemeal cereals have the effect of balancing the immune system as a whole, harmonising the individual allergic reactions.

Apart from the acute cases, which should be treated and, if possible, their causes identified, there are chronic illnesses in which food allergies and intolerances may play an important role, such as childhood atopic dermatitis; reducing or eliminating some foods can often have considerable benefits.

An educative diet
The latest studies confirm what we anthroposophists have been upholding for over half a century, that is, too early a diversification of a neonate's diet facilitates the manifestation of an inherited tendency to allergies. In the very earliest period of life, the intestinal mucosa has still not acquired its characteristics of immunological protection against proteins other than those of maternal milk. The early introduction of a varied diet is, therefore, questionable.

Ice-cream and sweets proffered to babies only a few months old are a source of early sensitisation and allergic reactions to egg proteins, cow's milk and more.

Viral infections accentuate the natural fragility of the intestinal mucosa of infants; in the three weeks following an infection it is essential not to introduce new types of food.

Given that this is fundamentally a problem of life-style and general care, there are some remedies useful for allergic children. We mention them only to give an idea of the scope of the anthroposophic approach to allergies.

Conchae. Besides prophylactic calcium which I usually prescribe for the first two years of life[28], *Conchae*, calcium carbonate from oysters, at a power from *D6* to *D30*, can be used as a remedy for the stolid allergic child, with delayed ossification and typical sweating of the head before falling asleep, this latter being a sign of difficult detachment of the nerve-sense pole in the night and its inadequate connection during the day. This is a child who actually never sleeps properly and, therefore, needs to spend more time in bed and is never completely awake. *Conchae*, a mineral extracted from oysters, that is, from an animal helps us to find a balance with the external world and to not exaggerate in our response to external stimuli, which is precisely the problem in allergies.

Quartz. Another great remedy is powdered *Quartz*, often given in the morning, coupled with the *Conchae* which is given in the evening.

One remedy wakes us up in the morning, the other helps us to fall asleep in the evening. *Quartz*, or *silicium dioxide*, is a great remedy for the nerve-sense system and facilitates correct re-engagement in the morning. Human beings have a complex metabolism of silicium, first revealed by Rudolf Steiner and now, after more than half a century, confirmed by biochemical research. Silicium is present in every part of the body that must deal with the outer world, from the intestinal mucosa to the skin. Every one of the major organs, such as the lungs, heart and bowel, has a covering (respectively, the pleura, pericardium and peritoneum), steeped with the forces of quartz: these forces help us to understand the difference between ourselves and the external world.

Plumbum D14 / Stannum D14 2:1;
Plumbum D14 / Stannum D14 1:2.

---

[28] It is worth taking a pause in the hot, summer period, when calcium preparations are not indicated.

One interesting constitutional remedy is *Plumbum D14 / Stannum D14* in its two formulations: one form is made of two parts of lead for one part of tin and is indicated for stolid, sluggish children, the other is made of one part of lead for two parts of tin and is excellent for lean, excitable children.

These metals stimulate the formative forces that start from the nerve-sense system, taking into account the constitution of the child or adolescent, in the case of asthma and rhinitis.

These are maintenance remedies with a very slow, but safe and effective action.

Treating to educate both humans and the world

The image that anthroposophic medicine offers us with regards to treating allergies, the principles for preventing them and even the remedies used can be summarised in an educational ideal: the treatment of allergies consists in a reconciliation with the world. A human being does not educate himself by reducing his dialogue with the world, nor by silencing dialogue with himself. This education is accomplished *not by desensitisation*, as a science that is a prisoner of nineteenth century molecular certainties would like us to believe, but, quite the contrary, it can be achieved by *humanisation*: I believe strongly that the "substance" of the world, passing through the human being has the possibility of evolving. When prescribing quartz, I am motivated by a medical desire to mitigate harm, but also by the certainty that the grains of quartz, with their capacity to absorb light, wait within the human body for yet more noble duties than their divine transparency.

It is divine to relieve suffering, but compassion and awareness are also divine: the soul becoming great through its reception of nature.

Hay fever

Hay fever, as mentioned in the previous chapter, is related to an allergic reaction to pollen which is manifested during the pollen season. This reaction is preceded by the pollen[29] penetrating the nasal, ocular and oropharyngeal mucosae. We have described how the body tries to remove alien substances by secretion, but with an exaggerated response and generating a local congestive inflammation and general symptoms.

We shall consider this illness taking into account the growing tendency to allergies in human beings in the twentieth century, and even more so in the twenty-first century; this changing tendency shows us that there has been an alteration in the relationship between the body and soul, between nature and man.

An ever increasing number of substances induce hypersensitivity. Immunology has made great progress towards understanding allergic phenomena, but for us it is also important to understand what forces are involved in an allergic reaction. It is worth going beyond the technicalities, albeit important, of the encounter between the external enemy, the *antigen*, represented by the pollen, and the *antibody*, the internal defender that acts in an exaggerated way.

Observing the phenomenon without preconceptions we realise that Rudolf Steiner was right when he taught that an allergic reaction is caused *more by the seasonal environmental stimulus than by the pollen* suspended in the air, as shown by the typical *allergic crises at wakening,* even before having opened the windows. The pollen is the same, but the stimuli, such as light, colour and temperature, are increased.

Our excessive response is unleashed with the deafening rhythm of our war drums: bursts of sneezing.

[29] Substances that penetrate into the body and provoke an allergic reaction are called *antigens* or *allergens*. In the case of hay fever, pollens are the allergens, but allergic rhinitis can be caused by many other respiratory allergens, such as various types of animal fur and dust-mites.

In hay fever there is a predisposition of our astral body, our soul, to lose itself, to imitate the corresponding process of the external world; this makes the astral body less efficient within the body, in the metabolism, in performing its task of separating, controlling and humanising external substances according to the instructions of the "I". The result of this is that, with the arrival of the spring in which everything prospers in the liquid element, the decreased activity of the astral body in the metabolism enables excessive secretory activity of the etheric and an upward aqueous swelling: a general swamping of the mucous membranes of the head. The patient does not dominate the fluid body and excessive excretion appears in inappropriate sites.

There are two aspects that are evident.

The first is *an incapacity to control the water body*.

Sufferers from hay fever have a clinical history of an *exudative diathesis*, typical of children who sweat profusely, particularly from the head, and suffer from "lymphatism", an excessive production of tissue lymph that impairs growth and vitality. Such children are often sluggish and apathetic.

The other aspect is the *excessive permeability of the nasal mucous membranes to grass pollens*.

The pollens penetrate untransformed into the mucous membranes and promote an allergic reaction. This increased permeability expresses a general, and not only local, inability to defend the boundaries of our inner world from external life. Delayed defences and an inflammatory reaction are related to the release of histamine. Conventional medicine acts precisely on this last stage by using anti-histamines or corticosteroids to block the allergic reaction that causes the inflammation.

Apart from the known secondary effects of these drugs, such as drowsiness, we believe that acting at the end of this process prevents a full understanding of the illness and the identification of means to "educate" the body in its relationships with nature and with its own existential adventure.

We would like to highlight what we could call the *excessive stimulus to dilute*. We are thinking about the symptoms of allergy, with the rising tide of internal water, with the increased permeability of the mucosal membranes and the consequent excessive excretion: this is the state responsible for the marked sensitivity to pollen in people with hay fever.

The body's metabolic functions, flooded by fluid, lose the formative and limiting action of the organization of the "I" and in this context escape its control.

The watery inflammatory processes are a unilateral expression of the ether body, which has a particular relationship with the fluid body of the human being.

In hay fever, the ether body floods the mucosa with fluid, without there being the moderating effect of the astral body. There is an invasion of the metabolic processes such that these exceed their limits and invade the nerves and senses with a centrifugal force, i.e., a force towards the exterior, just as occurs contemporaneously in nature in the dynamics of dispersion of pollen that, released from the flower (which represents the metabolic sphere of the plant), saturates the atmosphere.

When a human being mimics the processes of nature, we have a pathological state; in fact, it is man's task to harmoniously overcome nature's processes within himself, and not to be dominated by them.

Citrus/Cydonia is a remedy for hay fever. The general treatment that we use in anthroposophic medicine for hay fever is based on the principle of thickening the liquid contained in the human body in order to make it denser and promote the reabsorption of substances into solution. In other words, it acts on the astral body, helping it to enter and constrain the ether body[30], restoring control of the metabolism and limiting its physical expansion, manifested by the swelling, oedema and congestive inflammation of the mucosal membranes of the eyes, nose and throat. We

---

[30] We act on the astral body in order to constrain the ether body dynamically, without damaging its vitality, without suppressing the body's action, replacing it as anti-histamines do, or weakening the defences as cortisone does.

search for the opposite process in nature, the process that we lack, the flower that does not bloom in "our garden".
Steiner indicated fruits with a leathery peel, in particular lemon and quince, as remedies.
Observing these it can be seen that they have a moulding force that acts from the outside inwards. We all know the strongly astringent property of lemon juice[31].
Its taste can be experimented directly or by observing the amusing grimaces of a child who tastes it. The hardness of its rind, its leathery form, can be appreciated when the fruit is left for a long time until it becomes dry: then the rind becomes hard! You need a sharp knife to open it and inside you will find pure lemon juice: the pulp present in the fresh fruit, and even more so in the unripe one, has been used up and pure juice remains in the centre. This separation of the pure liquid from the peel is the centripetal therapeutic action that we are looking for, the effect that makes the peel ever harder and the liquid ever denser.
The quince fruit is also surprising for its hardness; the soft, enchanted garden of the rose family contains peaches, plums, cherries and that apple, so full of flavour as to have cost us paradise! The quince is not edible in its natural state, but if it is cooked, continuing the desiccating work of the sun, together with sugar, crystallised light, then a delicious, dense syrup is obtained. This syrup is used from Sicily to Scandinavia to prepare quince jam or jelly, which is so thick that it takes the shape of the attractive moulds in which it can be placed. The setting power of pectin[32] causes *gelification*, an intermediate state between solid and liquid which once again expresses this "gesture" of thickening a liquid. Of course, here we are only interested in emphasizing the dominant idea behind the prescription of the typical remedy for hay fever, *Citrus/Cydonia*, consisting of lemon juice (*Citrus limon, succus*) and quince fruit extract (*Cydonia oblonga, fructus*). This

---

[31] Astringent: a substance that causes constriction.
[32] *Pectin* is a substance present in apples and is used as a thickener, for example to set jam after it has been boiled only very briefly.

remedy is useful for activating the astral body in relation to the etheric, before nature stimulates "our garden" too strongly to grow and soak up water. With the astringent effect of lemon juice, the astral body dominates the etheric liquid, while the minerals contained in the fruits' juices, such as potassium, calcium and silicium, support the organization of "I", which in its turn, sustains and stabilises the work of the astral body.

Citrus/Cydonia is administered into the body by subcutaneous injection, or applied externally as eye drops or nasal cream, or given by inhalation.

Clinical tests have demonstrated the extraordinary utility of this remedy, which in adults is injected, in increasing doses, between the shoulder blades before the pollen season; the inhalation route of administration is preferred in children, in order to avoid injections.

This background therapy must always be associated with a strictly personal treatment chosen by a punctilious doctor. Such a therapy must treat the causes of the illness and is difficult but usually resolves the problem.

Allergic conjunctivitis
Citrus/Cydonia eye drops are really an excellent help in the allergic conjunctivitis that accompanies hay fever. If these drops cause burning, which can occur in the case of dry eyes or in children, before adding them to the eyes, instil one of two drops of *Euphrasia D3 eye drops,* which reduce the acidity of the *Citrus/Cydonia* drops and moisten the eyes.

Symptomatic remedies
Euphrasia D3 drops. This is one of the main remedies for hay fever characterized by intense conjunctivitis with such profuse, irritant and excoriating lacrymal secretions as to redden the skin around the eyes, swollen, burning eyelids, red, painful eyes, photophobia, copious, non-irritant nasal secretions, little sneezing, disturbed breathing and a cough. The dose is 10 drops in a little water, every two or three hours, in adults and 4 to 7 drops in chil-

dren. This remedy is often used in association with eye drops.

Cepa D3 drops. This remedy is the polar remedy of the previous one. *Cepa D3 drops* are indicated when the symptoms comprise abundant nasal secretions (which soak a handkerchief) which are irritant enough to redden the skin around the nostrils and upper lip, a copious, non-irritant watery discharge from the eyes, and frequent, violent, "barrages" of sneezing. The symptoms are worsened by heat and improve with fresh air. The dose of *Cepa D3 drops* is similar to that of the *Euphrasia drops.* In cases in which the spasmodic crisis is very similar to that just described, it is worth using a higher dilution of the remedy, for greater efficacy; the dilution should, however, be prescribed by a doctor. In mixed forms in which both the eyes and the nose are irritated, the two remedies, *Cepa* and *Euphrasia*, can be alternated every two to three hours.

Sabadilla D4 drops. This is the third symptomatic remedy, which is valid in the case of repeated and particularly violent sneezing with spasmodic choking, nasal discharge and abundant tears, albeit not very irritating, sensitivity to the scent of flowers and lively itching of the throat, particularly the vault of the palate with a consequent desire to scratch the soft palate with the tongue. In these cases, the symptoms worsen with cold and improve with fresh air. The treatment is 10 drops every three or four hours, with the dose reduced to 5-7 drops in children.

Ribes Nigrum 1D gems, glycerol macerate. This is an interesting remedy that is not part of the anthroposophic tradition. It is made from blackcurrant buds and is a good background remedy for allergic tendencies; it is considered a natural stimulant of endogenous[33] production of cortisone. From an anthroposophic perspective, we appreciate its particular ability to stimulate the renal system and, above all, the adrenal system[34], increasing the

---

[33] *Endogenous* in medicine means produced by the body itself. Cortisone is produced in the adrenal glands and secreted into the blood.

[34] The adrenal glands are the site of stress-related processes, as we shall see in the chapter on asthma.

Hay fever

effectiveness of the constraint of the ether body by the astral body starting from below. In this context it provides a complementary action to *Citrus*, which curbs the ether body from above. Its draining action[35] is particularly useful in subjects clogged with anti-histamines, when the mucosal membranes of the nose are altered and obstructed by vasoconstrictive nasal drops, slowing the work of *Citrus*. The dose is 30-50 drops two or three times a day in a generous amount of water. This remedy has a valid preventive effect if taken one or two months before the start of the pollen season, but, at the same doses it also acts in the period of allergies. It is a treatment that can also be used in children, in which case the dose should be reduced to 20-25 drops in the morning and evening.

---

[35] In natural medicine the term used to describe the action of detoxifying and freeing the body of toxic compounds and harmful waste is *drainage*.

Asthma

"Submit to being called a neurotic. You belong to that splendid and pitiable family which is the salt of the earth. All the greatest things we know have come to us from neurotics. It is they and they only who have founded religions and created great works of art. Never will the world be conscious of how much it owes to them, nor above all of what they have suffered in order to bestow their gifts on it. We enjoy fine music, beautiful pictures, a thousand exquisite things, but we do not know what they cost those who wrought them in sleeplessness, tears, spasmodic laughter, rashes, asthma" (Marcel Proust).

Asthma is related to wakeful consciousness
In patents with asthma the difficulty in breathing increases with the simple fact of being awake, of feeing observed or of wanting to attract attention. Sometimes it seems that the patient unconsciously plays with his own illness. The astral body and organization of "I" rhythmically abandon the physical-ether body with the passage into sleep and re-enter it on awakening. We can understand how asthma arises from an altered relationship between the soul and life, between the astral body and the physical-ether body. The psychological symptoms of asthmatic patients are very complex and multifaceted. It is clear that asthma can be worsened by psychological factors, but also that it can be improved by sedation as well as by "compassion"[36], an experience that ennobles the art of medicine. In asthma, the astral body places an obstacle to exhalation that starts from the ether body, the expirato-

---

[36] We obviously mean an *objective compassion*, free of emotion or sentimentalism, based on an effective understanding. Objective compassion founded on the knowledge of the human being creates an attitude of the soul which enters the whole human being and does not rest a prisoner of sentiment. Sentimental compassion incorporates a sort of humiliating pity that should be rejected (see Rudolf Steiner, *The Healing Education Course* (CW 317), from a conference on 26/06/1924).

Asthma

ry flow is entrapped in the astral body, slows down and is blocked. The illness does not have external causes, the obstacle lies with the patient himself, in his astral body.

This makes the patient resistant to treatment and the illness difficult to cure. Rudolf Steiner rightly defined asthma a *"refined illness"*. Although asthma is manifested in the lungs, its real roots are where the air body is regulated, i.e., in the renal system, which includes the adrenal glands. If a person is under tension for any reason, the adrenal glands produce various reactions described by Selye as stress. Stress is an expression of an excessive and continuous hold by the astral body, which is manifested by increased vigilance, blood pressure and blood sugar levels and, which if prolonged, can lead to illness. The astral body is the carrier of the forces of illness, just as the ether body is the carrier of the forces of healing. Health is a dynamic state, a continuous equilibrium between constructive etheric forces and destructive astral ones.

In asthma there are *spasms,* an activity of the astral body that has not been incorporated correctly. The kidney is not diseased, but renal function is disturbed. "The essential conventional therapeutic components are corticosteroids"[37], cortisones, but also ephedrine and adrenaline, all drugs aimed at treating the renal (kidney-adrenal gland) system. In homeopathy a fundamental medicine for the treatment of asthma is *Cuprum*, copper, the metal related to the forces of Venus, the cosmic archetype of renal function. *Theophylline*, a drug typically used to treat asthma, works through the kidneys, promoting diuresis. Even the bland diuretic action of caffeine can help an asthmatic.

Notions regarding treatment

Physiologically at night the astral body separates from the physical-etheric body to induce sleep. In asthma, however, the astral body is *imprisoned* in the lungs; the strategy, therefore, is to support the descent of the astral body, returning it to the kidneys

---

[37] *Medical Letter*, year XXIX, n. 8, 15 April 2000.

and, thereby, breaking its pathological link with the lungs. The administration of inhaled corticosteroids is advantageous because of the anti-inflammatory effects of these compounds, but they are only a symptomatic treatment: the asthma remains. Symptomatic treatment is fundamental, and truly integrated modern medicine must recognize this: during attacks we can use conventional treatments. However, the real task of medicine is to prevent an attack from recurring. We must treat the person in the intervals between the attacks, not in the acute phase. We must push the astral body into the kidneys, not just detach it from the lungs as cortisone does. Steiner considered that a general characteristic of an asthmatic was his lack of appropriate boundaries: the asthmatic is permeable to emotions just as he is permeable to changes in the weather, with his condition worsening with dampness.

In order to show you the breadth of anthroposophic care, we would like to mention a treatment that is of course used under prescription from a doctor. This treatment consists of a very interesting sequence of three remedies that are injected in three different areas of the body. The first remedy is *Prunus spinosa*, a plant that stimulates the ether body. It is injected into the area of the nape of the neck: carrying etheric forces into the nerve-sense pole, which is enlivened, i.e. the downwards movement of the astral body is promoted. *Citrus medica/Cydonia*, the main remedy of hay fever, is injected in the area between the shoulder blades and has the purpose of thickening and densifying the body's fluids. *Nicotiana tabacum*, a very astral, poisonous plant, which draws the astral body downwards, is injected in the area of the kidneys.

The treatment is effective if the injections are given on alternate days. This rhythm also corresponds to the different actions: the upper region is vivified, while in the central area the astral body must be attracted inwards and then finally drawn down with the poison (astral stimulus) to the renal system. In children and individuals extremely sensitive to injections, the treatment can be given in the form of *inhalations*. An ointment of copper in substantial form and potentized tobacco (*Cuprum/Tabacum*), applied

and massaged daily over the kidneys, is also useful. Ointments are the modern, anthroposophic equivalent of acupuncture, but unlike acupuncture, in which the patient is passive, the use of ointments requires active participation by the patient. The oral route of administration can be used to avoid injections, particularly in children, but also as an auxiliary to the injected therapy:
Quercus cortex D1 drops in the morning,
Veronica officinalis D1 drops in the evening.
Oak bark is rich in tannins, astringent substances that help the astral body enter the organs of metabolism. Speedwell can be seen in the summer in meadows and with its sky blue-violet flowers recalls copper and Venus; this remedy promotes the sense of harmony and peace that humans need to be able to release the astral body and "I" when falling asleep. It is useful for patients with bronchial catarrh who cannot get to sleep because of impellent coughing. This dual therapy promotes order and harmony in the astral body and can be considered an extension of *Nicotiana*, which could be given in the form of an ointment. It is not uncommon that this treatment alone is sufficient in children not being treated with synthetic drugs.
Cichorium Plumbo cultum D2 drops. This is a remedy particular to anthroposophic medicine, which uses herbal remedies, such as chicory, the main plant in the treatment of hepatobiliary function in children: it supports digestive activities, helps against dyspepsia and fermentation and is also useful for constipation. It is essential to support the liver during an allergic illness, because this organ plays a central role in the metabolism of proteins. In allergies there is a decrease in the activity of the astral body and hyperactivity of the ether body in the site affected (in fact, there is always an element of overflowing liquids, both in rhinitis and in the blisters occurring in dermatitis) and, on the other hand, in the liver there is astral hyperactivity and a weakness of the ether body. Thus, supporting the liver means helping it in its function of perceiving the quality of the substances that enter the body from the outside world.
We can make *Cichorium* a yet better ally of the liver if we grow it

Part II. Illnesses and remedies

in earth that has been sprinkled with lead, which has an affinity with hepatogastric digestion starting from the spleen, the great balancer of the process of perceptive digestion. The spleen plays an essential role in supporting the immune system. Indeed, one of the most feared complications of splenectomy (the surgical removal of the spleen) is a marked susceptibility to infections; another complication is acute intestinal blockage. Having observed some of my splenectomised patients[38], I believe that a few drops of this remedy can have such a marvellous effect precisely because the plant does not absorb lead, but rather its dynamics. Given that it is the permeability of the mucous membranes that makes an allergy severe, the efficacy of this remedy lies in the fact that it prevents exactly this process.

In small children this remedy is used in cycles, in order not to overstimulate the children through the stimulatory effect of vegetabilised lead on the nervous system.

I do urge that, as for all maintenance treatments, a medical prescription is needed for this remedy. The same holds true for the other interesting remedy, which is:

Equisetum arvense Silicea cultum D2 drops.

The horsetail can be considered a "kidney" plant *par excellence*. It forms saponins that recall the connection – evident in the formation of foam – between the astral-air and the etheric-water. Furthermore, the plant, which is extremely rich in silicium, has a real quartz skeleton. In human beings it increases the sensitivity of the kidneys and supports their activity. The plant grown for this medicinal preparation is given a quartz fertiliser that accentuates its relationship with the distinctive quality of the kidneys. Supporting the kidneys means lightening the work of the nerve-sense system in the periphery of the body, be it in the skin or in the mucosal membranes. This remedy is a useful aid in inflammatory renal disorders, in skin disorders and in diseases such as asthma in which there is excessive neurosensory activity in the periphery of the body.

---

[38] That is, they have had their spleen removed surgically.

The challenge of asthma

The diagnosis of asthma is complex and requires an understanding of the other systems of the body involved in order to choose the non-medicinal accompanying treatments. It demands humility on the part of the doctor and compels him to work with other doctors and therapists. Nowadays one would say that it requires a multidisciplinary approach. We prefer to say that it requires the support of a therapeutic community in which the doctor assumes his responsibility and does not hide behind specialists. *Rhythmical massage*[39] is appropriate; other very useful treatments are *eurythmy therapy*[40], *anthroposophic magnetotherapy, lemon compresses* and the *application of copper* in various ways, as we have already indicated regarding the ointment in the previous paragraph. *Anthroposophic art therapy*[41] is of fundamental help in this process of inner growth that is the treatment of asthma. It could be said that this illness requires that the doctor acts as a "midwife", enabling and empowering the patient's participation; asthma also becomes an extraordinary occasion for the moral growth of a doctor. This is seen precisely in the case in which there seems to be a clinical failure: the miracle may then occur that the fickle

---

[39] The *Hauschka rhythmical massage* is a specific type of massage used in anthroposophic medicine and which has interesting therapeutic principles.

[40] *Eurythmy*, or the "visible word", is a complex discipline of movement which offers the possibility of using the limbs to express the etheric reality of the human movement that starts from the larynx, an organ fundamentally involved in exhalation. Eurythmy therapy is one of the jewels of anthroposophic curative arts and can be used in various disorders, from short-sightedness to scoliosis, and in the treatment and prevention of hypertension.

[41] *Art therapy* started in the 1920s from the collaboration between Rudolf Steiner, the founder of anthroposophy, and Dr. Ita Wegman, who was a pioneer of anthroposophic medicine. Dr. Hauschka, one of Ita Wegman's colleagues, was the first to apply art therapy, which she then taught for many years in the school in Boll in Germany. The main disciplines are watercolour painting, sculpting and drawing, flanked by eurythmy, developed predominantly through the dedication of Steiner's wife, Marie von Sivers. Nowadays there are schools of both art therapy and eurythmy in various countries. Only after a long and complex training, including practical experience in an anthroposophic medical setting, can one practise as an anthroposophic art therapist or eurythmy therapist.

modern human being becoming a faithful, trusting patient who returns repeatedly to the doctor, helping him overcome the mechanistic temptation to consider the persistence of the patient's asthma as a clinical failure. Goethe, the great poet, scientist and forerunner of anthroposophy, described this in a wonderful way:
"In the act of breathing there are two gifts of grace:
one oppresses, the latter refreshes.
And so life is wondrously mixed!
Thank you God when you burden us
and thank you when you set us free again".

Considerations on the acute phase of the illness
Asthma is a chronic inflammatory disorder of the airways characterized by a state of non-specific hyper-reactivity of the bronchi, which is manifested by bronchial obstruction, almost always reversible, with the clinical signs of difficulty in breathing, cough and wheezing. Once this situation has developed, it is self-perpetuating and self-amplifying. The worsening local inflammation and obstruction underlie the hyper-reactive state of the affected mucous membranes. It is becoming ever clearer that asthma is the sum of various events with a complex and multifactorial pathogenesis[42] and develops on a genetic disposition that conditions its varied expression.

From an aetiological perspective asthma is a heterogeneous disorder. There are many stimuli that can trigger acute episodes, but it is worth describing two particular types of asthma: allergic asthma and intrinsic or idiosyncratic asthma.

Allergic asthma is by far the more frequent, accounting for about 80% of cases of asthma. Atopy is the main risk factor for the development of this type of asthma. Allergic asthma is often associated with a personal and/or family history of allergic disorders such as rhinitis, urticaria and atopic dermatitis.

People with atopy have an exaggerated response, characterized

---

[42] Pathogenesis: a process or mechanism of developing an illness.

by the production of immunoglobulin E (IgE) antibodies against specific allergens, both inhaled and ingested with food, by high levels of total serum IgE, skin tests positive to allergenic extracts, and positive tests with specific challenges. The quality of the immune response by the T lymphocytes seems to depend on both genetic and environmental factors. The onset of asthma in children is favoured by the concentration of inhaled allergens in the environment, by some viral respiratory tract infections, by scarce and altered bacterial intestinal flora, by the type of diet in the early years of life, by active and passive tobacco smoke (both inhaled directly and from the surroundings), by industrial pollution and it has been discovered recently that asthma is also more common in people who have not had infections such as measles, primary tuberculosis (a benign, asymptomatic form occurring in childhood) and hepatitis A. These factors, alone or in combination, can alter the regulatory immune mechanisms of the mucous membranes, such as to cause an allergenic-based inflammatory response mediated by particular types of lymphocytes. Once a subject is sensitised, contact with even a small amount of the allergen is sufficient to trigger the chain of events that leads to allergic inflammation. This reaction occurs immediately in all cases, while 30-50% of subjects also have a subsequent later stage (6-9 hours after contact with the allergen) which resolves slowly. Various studies, including official ones, have been published. The results of a Swedish study, published in the prestigious, mainstream medical journal "The Lancet"[43] are famous.

---

[43] "Lancet", 1999, 353: 1485-1488, Alm J.S., Swartz J., Lilja G., Scheynius A., Pershagen G., *Atopy in children with an anthroposophic lifestyle*. In a study published in the "The Lancet", carried out in children who attended Waldorf schools, it was seen that the incidence of allergies was notably lower than that in the general population. The study involved 295 children, aged between 5 and 13 years old, who went to two Waldorf schools in Stockholm (Sweden) and 380 other children of the same age who were brought up with conventional life-style and diet. The researchers considered any history of atopy, the frequency of infectious diseases, use of antibiotics, vaccination and social and environmental factors. It was found that 52.5% of the children in the Waldorf schools had received antibiotics in the past, compared with 90% of the children in the other group; 18%

This study showed that there was a lower incidence of allergies and asthma among pupils at Waldorf schools than among pupils attending normal schools. It does, therefore, seem clear that the aim of asthma treatment should be to control the chronic inflammatory state that underlies the illness and that it not necessary to wage war, out of principle, with the acute phase. In the absence of a quick improvement in response to anthroposophic remedies, the patient should be treated with mainstream medicines. The patient, or his mother, usually learns to distinguish allergic crises of different severity.

An acute asthma attack is not the occasion for amateur anthroposophic home care. If a doctor cannot be present, recourse should be made to traditional treatments which, in the acute phase, are essentially bronchodilators and steroids. These are important drugs in an acute emergency. The use of inhaled prod-

in the Waldorf schools had been given the trivalent measles-mumps-rubella vaccine, compared to 93% of the other children, while 63% of the children in the Waldorf schools had only been vaccinated against measles. Vegetables containing lactobacilli were eaten by 63% of the children attending the Waldorf schools and by only 4-5% of those in the control group. Skin tests and blood tests showed that the children in the Waldorf schools had a lower prevalence of atopy compared with the other children. It could, therefore, be concluded that there is a proportional, inverse relationship between the main features of a healthy, anthroposophic lifestyle and the risk of atopy. We briefly describe another very interesting scientific study: "Lancet", 2001, 358, 1129-33, *Exposure to farming in early life and development of asthma and allergy: a cross-sectional survey*. In numerous studies carried out in children in Sweden, Switzerland, Finland, Austria and Bavaria, a lower incidence of allergic phenomena was found in children living in rural areas than in those living in the city. Most of the research cited was performed in Austria, where 2283 children aged 8 to 10 years old were studied, of whom 1137 underwent skin tests for seven local allergens. Simplifying the findings, we can say that children who lived in the countryside had a lower incidence of hay fever and asthma, despite being more exposed to pollen and allergy-provoking substances. This phenomenon is explained in various ways: for example, it could be due to the development of immune tolerance or to a resetting of the immune balance because of the greater exposure of children in the countryside to microbes, in particular, according to some researchers, the mycobacteria and actinomycetes found in farms and fields. It was found that untreated, not boiled milk does not provoke allergies and actually reduces the risk of asthma.

ucts, improvements in pre-dosed inhalers, the introduction of spacers, new non-chlorofluorocarbon propellants and dry powders without propellants have all led to versatile, easily used systems requiring lower doses of drugs and, thereby, reducing the side effects of these treatments. You should not, therefore, be shocked if an anthroposophic doctor prescribes traditional remedies in the acute phase. I myself sometimes use a combination of anthroposophic remedies and synthetic drugs with great benefit. For example, we can reduce the dose of bronchodilator needed in an aerosol to only two or three drops if we combine it with an appropriate anthroposophic remedy for the acute attack. This remedy could be a vial of *Nicotiana* in the case of spasmodic asthma or a vial of *Levico*, which contains arsenic, iron and copper, in the case of a dry cough and agitation, but also *Tabacum Cupro cultum* to combine tobacco and copper, or *Prunus* when the patient seems very weak. Symptomatic remedies taken orally can be useful if taken immediately the first symptoms appear. Subsequently, the classical remedies for allergy can be used, such as *Arsenicum album D30 drops*, which is useful, in frequent doses, for the treatment of an incessant dry cough which worsens towards the evening, various copper-based preparations, which are excellent anti-spasmodic treatments, such as *Cuprum D6* injected in the area of the kidneys or taken by aerosol, *Cuprum D6* powder administered every hour or half hour, and *Tabacum Cupro cultum*, in drops, vials or aerosol.

Other excellent remedies are *footbaths at increasing temperature* for children and *mustard footbaths* for adults, which can often resolve an attack of asthmatic bronchitis. For children, a very good treatment in the case of bronchitis, after a cold or when there is persistent cough, mucus or catarrh, is a *poultice of ricotta* on the chest. A poultice also has mucolytic and spasmolytic effects in the case of spasmodic asthmatic bronchitis. A piece of cotton 20 centimetres high, folded in two to form a pocket, and long enough to surround the circumference of the child's chest, is filled with a layer of ricotta (at room temperature) about one centimetre thick. This ricotta-filled pocket is placed on a terry towel folded length-wise which is then wrapped round the chest of the child, who will be in contact with the ricotta through the cotton cloth. The poultice should be kept in place for at least an hour and if it is applied in the evening, it can be kept for the whole night. The patient will sleep better because the mucus gradually loosens and coughing decreases, which enables lost sleep to be recovered. Another excellent remedy is *Lobelia comp. vial*, given either by injection or by aerosol: this is effective in re-balancing the neurosensory component, acting against the spasms and tachycardia often resulting from excessive use of bronchodilators.

As we have tried to show, the treatment of asthma focuses on the contrast between inner and outer worlds and so must be based on a global approach to the person and his way of facing existence. We must not miss this opportunity to treat the individual, taking into account that in a certain sense extreme schematism of a dominant treatment can imprison the individual into a stereotype leading to his illness becoming chronic. We can say that an asthmatic patient treated traditionally, with only symptomatic treatment, will remain asthmatic for the whole of his life. This is partly because some of the drugs used enter into daily life and slowly expel the body's capacity to react individually, according to its own needs, as occurs in the case of prolonged use of steroids and bronchodilators: the convenience of treatments does, therefore, risk preventing true healing. Indeed, all researchers working in this field agree in saying that although much progress has been made in understanding the pathophysiological mechanisms of asthma and, in consequence, its therapy, the classical drugs used, such as steroids, bronchodilators, chromones and antileukotrienes are not able to resolve the treatment and understanding of the illness completely. In this perspective, the enormous breadth of the anthroposophic approach is an opportunity to deal with the complexity of the asthmatic patient: a breath of air!

Conjunctivitis: the weeping eye

The conjunctiva is a mucous membrane that lines the internal surface of the eyelids and the anterior surface of the bulb of the eye, stopping at the cornea. Its task is to protect the eyelids and eyes from external agents and distribute tears in order to keep the surface of the eye clean and lubricated. Inflammation of the conjunctiva is called "conjunctivitis" and is one of the most common disorders of the eye. Various pathogens, such as viruses, fungi and bacteria, as well as toxic and allergic factors, can lead to the development of this inflammation which is manifested by some symptoms shared by all the types and others that are typical of the particular pathogen implicated.
The most common sign in all cases of conjunctivitis is reddening, with the internal surfaces of the eyelids and the bulb of the eye being most strongly affected. The catarrhal forms of conjunctivitis, typical in early infancy, are characterized by the presence of a mucus secretion that thickens along the rims of the eyelids. Almost always there is reddening of the skin at the edges of the eyelids, and involvement of the eyelashes. The bacteria can reach the conjunctiva in two ways: from the outside, through the air, dust, water or direct contact with the hands; and from the inside, rising up through the lacrymal canal and lacrymal sac.

Conjunctivitis in the neonate
One particularly important form of this eye condition is "gonococcal conjunctivitis of the neonate", which occurs by contagion at delivery as the neonate passes through the vagina. This disorder, which is of notable clinical importance because of the severe complications that it can cause, is due to an infection in the birth canal. The treatment is medical and is challenging.

Bacterial conjunctivitis
The bacterial forms of conjunctivitis are characterized by a variably intense redness of the conjunctiva, which changes colour

from pink to red. The tissue thickens and small haemorrhages occur. Swelling of the eyelids and redness of the surrounding skin indicate a more severe form: in this case a doctor must be consulted. A constant finding in bacterial forms of conjunctivitis is a muco-purulent secretion that collects at the rim of the eyelids, making it difficult to open the eyes on awakening. These cases of conjunctivitis are very frequently bilateral because of indirect contagion from one eye to the other; the child must be prevented from touching his eyes, great care must be taken with facial hygiene and contact with other children should be limited. Bacterial conjunctivitis requires a consultation with a doctor or, in the more severe cases, with an ophthalmologist. The description given here is intended to help recognition of the condition which always requires medical intervention.

Viral conjunctivitis

Viral conjunctivitis is associated with very abundant, clear tears and slight swelling of the eye (oedema). It requires medical care.

Allergic conjunctivitis

Allergic conjunctivitis is recognized from the marked swelling of the eyelids and the abundant, clear tears that irritate the skin around the eye and cause intense itching.

This condition has been dealt with in the chapter on hay fever.

Simple catarrhal conjunctivitis

There are various causes of irritation of the conjunctiva, including exposure to strong light, wind or dust, or the stress from reading or prolonged periods in front of a computer screen. Here are some typical remedies:

Euphrasia eye drops (contains *Euphrasia planta tota* D2 and *Rosa aetheroleum* D7);

Euphrasia D3 eye drops.

Instil one drop of one of the two remedies at a frequency ranging from twice a day to every two hours depending on the severity of the symptoms.

The eyebright (*Euphrasia*) that blooms in the summer in sun-flooded mountain meadows is the "image" of a healthy eye.
Eyebright calms and helps the functions of the eye and is, therefore, also useful in allergic conjunctivitis not only in the form of eye drops, but also as a remedy taken internally.
A warm, damp eye pack made with a *tea of chamomile* or, better still, *of fennel* and applied in the evening is always useful. After having filtered the tisane, wait until its temperature is acceptable, but do not allow it too cool too much, because a mild reddening of the eye due to the heat of the tisane promotes its soothing effect.
In the more acute forms in which the discharge begins to become turbid, a sign of bacterial proliferation, a few drops of *Calendula essence* can be added to the liquid used for the eye pack, while waiting to see a doctor.

Dry conjunctivitis
In the case of a dry, irritant conjunctivitis that causes reddening but scarce lacrymation use *Mercurialis eye drops*.
Instil one drop two or three times a day into the conjunctival sac. This remedy stimulates secretion from the eye glands. It contains etheric rose oil which has a harmonising effect.

Infections superimposed on allergic conjunctivitis
If the inflammation described in the allergies worsens, a mineral component, high potency rock crystal (quartz), should be added to the treatment. This effectively attenuates the metabolic processes that have been intensified by the disorder.
Echinacea/Quartz comp. eye drops should be used two or three times a day, instilling one drop into the conjunctival sac every two or three hours.
This remedy can be associated with a classical anti-inflammatory agent such as *Silicea comp. globules*, at a dose of 5 to 10 globules, to be dissolved in the mouth, every one, two or three hours; this treatment should not be suspended abruptly, but gradually tapered down as the symptoms improve.

Dacryocystitis and obstruction of the naso-lacrymal duct in neonates

Dacryocystitis is an inflammation of the lacrymal sac.

Chronic dacryocystitis may be manifested by tears alone; the *acute form* causes both lachrymation and secretions, with inflammation, tenderness, pain and swelling in the area of the lacrymal sac. A medical consultation is necessary.

Obstruction of the naso-lacrymal duct is very common in babies and it is useful if parents point out the problem to their doctor. The symptoms usually appear when the baby is about one to two months old and consist of tears and a chronic muco-purulent secretion in the affected eye. Usually only one eye is involved. Gentle massage of the lacrymal sac causing extrusion of purulent material from the tiny tear holes on the lower rim of the eye confirms the diagnosis.

If the symptoms persist the naso-lacrymal duct must be explored with a probe. This is indicated after nine to twelve months of age, given that many obstructions open spontaneously within one year of age. Gentle, warm, damp eye packs made with a *tisane of fennel* and applied in the evening, can help to overcome the milder forms and thereby the need for an intervention.

Sty

A sty is a small abscess of a gland on the edge of the eyelid and is usually caused by a staphylococcal infection. It generally occurs in debilitated subjects or as a consequence of conjunctivitis or inflammation of the eyelid. Warm, damp eye packs with *Calendula essence* are useful: dilute a teaspoon of the essence in a glass of hot water. Apply to the eye, taking care not to scald the area.

After the eye pack, spread *Mercurius vivus naturalis D5 ointment* around the eye and eyelids, using a gentle circular massage to help the absorption of the ointment.

Earache

In this chapter on earache, which in most cases is caused by otitis, we will focus mainly on children, in whom this disorder is particularly relevant. Good care of otitis in infancy is an occasion to strengthen the immune system as well as offering the possibility of a definitive resolution of the problem. Given the closeness of the anatomical structures in the nerve-sense pole, a cold or tonsillitis in a child can very easily give rise to *otalgia*, more commonly known as earache.

The pain develops because catarrh enters the middle ear and presses on the eardrum. Often this is only a transient part of the disorder and should not be dramatized. There is an extraordinarily good remedy which you may mock, but which I, without any presumption, suggest after more than twenty years of professional experience. This is an *onion poultice*, which is applied over the mastoid (the area behind and a little lower than the ear lobe). This has the function of "drawing out" the inflammation, soothing the pain and protecting against the feared complication of *mastoiditis* in a very reassuring way.

A raw onion is chopped up and put in the centre of a gauze (or cloth) which is then folded along the four sides and held closed with a sticking plaster to form a medicated compress. The compress is placed on the area behind the earlobe and fixed with a headscarf or elastic band around the head. It should be held in place for several hours and applied a few times a day. In the case of restless infants, a slice of onion can be fixed directly against the skin with a paper plaster. *I do not know of any other safer and more effective external treatment for otitis.*

It is worth repeating the application for several days, at least in the evening before going to bed, since lying down increases the pressure of the catarrh on the eardrum, which can cause the pain in the ear to recur. The onion poultice has the merit of being easy to prepare and can resolve earaches without having to use other remedies.

We must be grateful to the humble onion, which controls the process of exuberant sulphur, constraining it through its very precise form of repeated layers.

It is, therefore, sulphur (the *sulphur* of alchemy), a universal remedy for the metabolism of human beings, that is acting, but also the formative process that constrains it and pushes it back into the body.

The onion is a sovereign remedy when a process of inflammation must be overcome within the body, such as in the ear or in a joint, or when it is causing tendinitis (for example, of the wrist or elbow).

As a pain reliever, another possible remedy is intra-auricular application of *homemade clove oil*, that is, oil warmed (not fried!) with a clove of garlic cut into quarters; the oil is left to cool and then a few drops are instilled into the ear three or four times a day.

Levisticum 10% oil is an excellent remedy for intra-auricular use: it reduces pain and has an important anti-inflammatory effect. A few drops are used three or four times a day, plugging the ear with a bit of cotton wool to keep the drops within the ear.

In the case of a full-blown otitis, besides the *onion poultice* which remains indispensable we can use a background anthroposophic anti-inflammatory treatment, alternating the two remedies described for a sore throat with a remedy specific for the ear:

Apis D3 drops,
Belladonna D4 drops,
Levisticum D3 drops.

Apis and *Belladonna* are usually taken together, 3 to 6 drops of each into a small amount of water.

This mixture is alternated every two or three hours with *Levisticum*, 10 drops.

The dose for children can be reduced to 3 drops of *Apis D3* and 3 of *Belladonna D4*, alternated every two or three hours and to 5-7 drops of *Levisticum*. If the fever is high, the remedies can be alternated every hour.

Clinical experience has led me to prefer the alcoholic drops even in small children, because they are more effective and work more rapidly[44].

These drops are administered frequently, preferably every hour. Once the pain has been relieved, and perhaps also the fever, the dose is reduced to once every two hours, then once every three or four hours and continued, in the case of true otitis, for at least ten to twelve days. Otitis, once established, must be treated in depth, because the body has found an open access and uses it to create a focus of warmth in the head, which has cooled down and cannot dispose of the excessive catarrh deriving from the metabolism.

Here we mention only the strictly medical treatments, recalling that an episode of otitis always requires treatment by a doctor who, if he is an anthroposophist, will certainly appreciate your initial, personal intervention with the onion poultice and eardrops.

In the most challenging cases a nebuliser treatment can be give once or twice a day with:

Arnica/Levisticum D3 vial.

Quartz is another great anthroposophic remedy, although not recommended during the congestive phase because we need to see what happens to the eardrum. Thus, neither quartz nor high potency mercury-based preparations should be used without a prescription from your doctor, who will evaluate whether to thin the fluids or wait. The high potency homeopathic remedies, by thinning liquids too much and causing excessive drainage, can increase the risk of a burst eardrum, which is certainly an undesirable event.

Nevertheless, a *ruptured tympanic membrane* (burst eardrum) should not cause a drama: the fluids must be thinned well and

---

[44] Some anthroposophic doctors and paediatricians prefer the already described globules. We have: *Apis/Belladonna globules* and *Apis/Levisticum D2/D3 globules*, both specifically for earache. According to my colleagues, since these do not contain alcohol, their action is more appropriate for a child's body. This is a highly respectable point of view, even though I personally prefer a slightly more aggressive treatment based on alcohol.

then, after waiting a few days, closure of the perforated membrane should be promoted through the administration of a preparation of high potency quartz prescribed by your anthroposophic doctor, who you should contact for all cases of true otitis.

Echinacea
Echinacea tablets, described in the chapter on sore throat, are an excellent remedy for incipient otitis (as for all cold-related illnesses) both in the second stage of acute catarrhal otitis and subsequently to avoid recurrences. At the beginning of the problem, dissolve one tablet in the mouth every two or three hours (reduce the dose to half a tablet for children), then continue for several weeks, taking the tablets two or three times a day, both to strengthen the immune defences and to continue the fluidifying action and curative effect on the mucosae. The tablets have a very pleasant taste because they contain eucalyptus oil, a balsamic remedy *par excellence*.

Dental disorders

Toothache always requires the care of a dentist; the efficacy of anthroposophic treatments often ends up increasing our "laziness" and as soon as the pain diminishes, we forget all our good intentions. Since most dental problems need professional treatment, if we do not go quickly to the dentist, we risk damaging our precious dental apparatus. I do, therefore, urge you to go to the dentist regularly to prevent serious damage and, I may also say, avoid greater expenses.

Right from its start, anthroposophic medicine was interested in the teeth; certainly, many patients will already know *Rhatany toothpaste, Soluble saline toothpaste* and *Toothpaste for children*, all based on substances such as salt, myrrh, rhatany and calendula, which help the *prevention* of caries and are the result of a view of teeth as a sophisticated and complex organ that interacts with the whole body, particularly intellectual activity, the organs of movement and deliberate actions.

Already back in the nineteen-fifties a study showed that the incidence of dental caries was significantly lower in children attending Waldorf schools than in children going to traditional schools; in fact, dental caries is favoured by early intellectualism, an ultra-refined diet and limited or overly mechanical physical activity. Sugar, poor dental hygiene and unfortunate heredity should only be considered as second-line factors that favour tooth decay and damage to the gums and articulations of the dental apparatus.

Anthroposophic medicine offers treatments that are very useful for reducing the development of caries, so go regularly to your dentist for local prevention and treatment and to your anthroposophic doctor for general prevention and care. You will be satisfied.

Neuralgic tooth pain
A good remedy for neuralgic tooth pain of sudden onset due to lesions that inflame dental nerves is *Aconitum D8 drops*, 10 drops

every one, two or three hours in adults and from 3 to 7 drops in children.
This remedy relieves the inflammation of the nerves and enables the patient to endure the hours until going to the dentist. However, after some time, when the inflammatory process involves the structures around the tooth, it is no longer effective.
In the first stage, *Aconitum* can be combined with a slice of onion, applied whole to the cheek over the site of the painful tooth.
In the doubt that the inflammation has already involved the area around the root of the tooth, another useful remedy is *Aconitum comp. globules*, 10 globules every hour in adults or 7 globules every half hour; this remedy also contains belladonna, another great treatment in cases of inflammation.

Teething pains
This pain in the ear appears during teething in babies but can also be very intense in youngsters and adults when the molars or wisdom teeth break through. Steiner advised taking a *plantain leaf*, rolling it up and introducing it into the painful ear.
I limit myself to advising a tincture of *Plantago m.t.*: put one or two drops into a teaspoon of warm water and then pour the solution into the ear of the child, lying on his flank, wait for one or two minutes and then dry away any liquid that comes out of the ear. The drops of tincture can also be taken in a little water every three or four hours by mouth.
An alternative in less painful forms is *Aconitum comp. eardrops*; one drop of oil warmed to body temperature to instil in the ear from three to five times a day.

Pain caused by a dental abscess
Apis/Belladonna globules,
Apis D3 drops and *Belladonna D4 drops*.
These are the anti-inflammatory remedies *par excellence* of anthroposophic medicine, as described in the chapter on sore throat: the dose is 7 drops of both in half a cup of water or 10

globules dissolved in the mouth; this remedy is alternated every hour with:

Silicea comp. globules, 10 globules dissolved in the mouth. After two or three days, once the symptoms have improved, reduce the frequency of administration, alternating the two remedies every two hours for two or three days and then take it three or four times a day, for example *Silicea comp.* before the three meals and *Apis/Belladonna* after the three meals for another three to six days, while in the meantime having started dental treatment to resolve the inflammation and reduce the pain.

Sun-dried, fine green clay. This is very useful as a poultice to apply externally to the cheek: the clay powder is diluted with water and a teaspoon of olive oil is added to reduce the desiccant effect. A layer of a few centimetres of the resulting paste is applied externally over the site of the abscess, left in place for at least three quarters of an hour and then removed; the clay should not be reused.

Argiltubo green clay contains already prepared clay that can be applied directly. It is very useful when travelling or on holiday. Clay is a marvellous therapeutic resource whenever there is an inflammatory process or infection to control. Do not worry if the symptoms appear to worsen after applying the clay; this is not a bad sign, it is simply a transient effect due to increased circulation of blood within the site of the abscess. The blood carries white blood cells – lymphocytes and macrophages, warriors and scavengers of the evil.

This treatment can also be used for any superficial abscess *of the body, that is, for any collection of pus under the skin that is not serious enough to require surgical lancing.*

The real cure always passes through a small, critical moment which makes us aware of the greatness of the human condition: we are spiritual beings in an earthly vehicle which is also our noblest part; our angel helps us to endure toothache, but hopes that we experience that drop of infinity that sometimes hurts. The angel is not jealous because it is an angel, and knows that our physical pain is a noble promise for the future.

I have suffered from toothache very frequently. For long nights I have hoped that the pain would cease, but still I feel that this experience of consciousness belongs to me as a human being.

Inflammation of the dental pulp[45]

Inflammation of the dental pulp (pulpitis) is the most "surgical" of dental pains: it does not respond except perhaps transiently to synthetic painkillers, antibiotics are useless, and there is constant, localised pain that is worsened by thermal stimuli, particularly warmth: even only lukewarm food can aggravate it. Indeed, food of any sort, particular sweet foods, also worsen it. The world seems a really miserable place.

It is a pain, lodged in the facial bones, that has no promise of resolving. You need urgent help from the dentist, but this problem usually occurs at Christmas or Easter and so you must give thanks for those dental clinics that work year round: a few minutes of work with the drill for that marvellous, immediate benefit. You can then go to your own dentist for more in depth treatment.

Tooth extractions

Arnica planta tota D6 drops, 10 drops in a little water or directly into the mouth: if possible taken the night before the extraction and again just before going into the dentist's surgery. After the extraction take 10 drops every one or two hours to reduce the pain and facilitate healing, then decrease the frequency of use to every two or three hours and continue for at least four or five days.

Aconitum comp. globules may also be alternated with *Arnica* in cases in which the extraction was complicated: the dose is 10 globules every hour.

Gingivitis

Gingivitis is an inflammation of the gums and is usually related to the formation of plaque rich in bacteria beneath the gums and a

---

[45] Pulpitis or endodontitis is an inflammation of the dental pulp and can be acute or chronic; it is usually the consequence of caries.

periodontal pocket also teeming with bacteria. It can have deep-seated causes and I limit myself here to giving advice on how to reduce the inflammation.

Bolus Eucalypti comp. powder. This excellent powder made from white clay and anti-inflammatory remedies can be used for prolonged mouthwashes and gargles. Put a level teaspoon of the powder into a glass of warm water, keep the solution covered in the bathroom and stir it every time before a mouthwash, which should be performed at least three or four times a day.

Activated green clay. This is sun-dried, breeze-ventilated clay appropriate for internal use; in fact it is used for all treatments involving oral intake of clay diluted in water. A heaped teaspoonful is put into a glass of water and stirred well; it can be used for prolonged mouthwashes and gargling three or four times a day, remembering to stir it every time before use. In order to reduce inflammation, it is useful to add a few drops of *Calendula essence* to the diluted clay.

In the most acute forms of gingivitis, use anti-inflammatory treatment with *Apis/Belladonna*, as already described for dental abscesses: you can also add *Calendula D3 drops*, 10 drops alternated every hour with *Apis/Belladonna* in drops or granules.

Cardiac antibiotic prophylaxis
Before undergoing any intervention to the mouth, patients with heart valves must start prophylactic antibiotic therapy; I do not consider it ethical to take chances in this situation.

Headache: when the head hurts

"*Time trieth truth*" (Thomas More).
We will try to describe this complex "system disease"[46] in a few lines, although it is undoubtedly too vast a subject to tackle in an introductory book on anthroposophic medicine. This disorder was long snubbed by medicine and by the chauvinism[47] which permeated the profession, being considered a sort of whim of elegant ladies; even the word migraine has a snobbish touch. The impressive increase in the incidence of headache has given support to a radically new point of view according to which this disorder is a sort of allergic response to internal bodily processes. Steiner, bringing a revolutionary new insight, indicated the cause of migraine as a digestive process that has "ascended" to the brain.

The brain is the central organ of the neurosensory system, but for its own nutritional processes, it needs a metabolism and a digestion; this need, in the case of a preponderant digestive process that rises from the metabolic zone and invades the brain, creates the foundations for pain, since the process finds itself in the wrong environment. Without an understanding of the functional trichotomy of humans it is difficult, if not impossible, to understand illnesses in which one functional complex of the body invades another. Conventional medicine has always tried to treat migraine and headache by acting on the nervous system (nerves

---

[46] It is beyond the scope of this book to give a classification of headaches, which range from classical migraine to cluster headaches; we only want to emphasize the functional bond connecting the three main functional systems of the human organization (nerve-sense, cardiorespiratory and metabolic-limb) whose dynamic equilibrium is disturbed. It is precisely this disturbance that leads to headache.
[47] One of the merits of anthroposophic medicine, which came about in response to a question from a female medical doctor, Ita Wegman, is that it has always had a strong female participation and leadership, even in times when women doctors were a rarity. This female presence in the movement can be recognised in the early interest of anthroposophic medicine in migraine and headache, in a period when traditional medicine paid hardly any attention to these problems.

and brain). Unfortunately, such treatment is only symptomatic since the real reasons for headache lie deep in the metabolism. The concept of a functional trichotomy helps the treatment of migraine greatly and explains the typical symptoms such as nausea and vomiting.

On this basis, Steiner gave the indications for a remedy which was called *"Biodoron"*, a compound based on silica, iron and sulphur, combined together using particular pharmaceutical processes. This remedy, specific for the treatment of migraine, is called *Ferrum-Quarz*. It exists in various formulations, so that the most appropriate one can be chosen by the doctor.

Quartz or silica facilitates the entry of the organization of "I" into the nerve-sense system; *sulphur* stimulates the forces in the metabolic sphere, activating metabolic processes in their specific environment and thereby withdrawing metabolic forces from the neurosensory pole; *iron* creates a rhythmic equilibrium between these two opposing stimuli, preventing the treatment leading to another one-sided imbalance, in other words, to a new illness.

Quartz is formed of silica and is transparent to light[48]. Silica is altruistic and a mediator and allows itself to be traversed by the spirit as such or as the creative principle from the environment. It makes what is earthly accessible to the cosmic creator. The action of silica as a substance is part of the nerve-sense system. However, as a process, as a dynamic action, silica enters the metabolic-limb system, where it enables synchronisation and the reciprocal perception of the organs. For this reason it is excreted in the urine as a substance.

On the other hand, a weak astral body, which connects inadequately with the ether body, can represent a barrier to the organization of "I", which can no longer influence the metabolism in a regulated way. Clinically, this can be manifested in functional alterations of the menstrual cycle, in which migraine attacks, which are difficult to resolve, are associated with menses.

---

[48] The silica that is used is quartz, a crystal, which allows light to pass through it.

Part II. Illnesses and remedies

Current thinking is so dominated by "fight the illness directly" that is difficult to understand the new concepts which require a complete review or at least a broadening of the way we look at headaches.

The side effects of drugs often originate from treating an illness in a one-sided manner, which simply results in another one-sided problem. When considering the preparation of remedies, Steiner drew on a concept already proposed by Goethe, imagining the production of a remedy as the creation of a *homunculus*, a little man who heals; the shape of this *homunculus* varies depending on the therapeutic impetus; in the *Ferrum-Quarz* remedy, we can imagine him with a generous belly and a large head, representing the site of the nerves and senses. In this remedy we have a connection between the three different substances from which it is made with each of the three parts of the trichotomous functional organization of the human being:

Nerve-sense system:	QUARTZ
Rhythmic system (cardiorespiratory):	IRON
Metabolic system:	SULPHUR

Steiner gave this little healing man, a harmonic *homunculus* materialised in the remedy, a significance that goes well beyond the treatment of migraine. In fact, we use this remedy for much broader purposes. For example, it is an excellent remedy for anaemia, in particular anaemia resulting from excessive intellectual activity, but also for mitigating a pregnancy-related anaemia, keeping the anaemia within the physiological range that occurs normally during pregnancy.

Even today we are struck by the "feats" of the so-called "archetypal" remedies of anthroposophic medicine, which are a sort of gift for organs or body functions. The most famous archetypal remedy is *Onopordon/Primula comp.*, whose real name is *Cardiodoron* ("doron", like donation, a gift, for the heart), which we have already discussed.

Headache: when the head hurts

Given the foregoing considerations, it is easy to understand that the treatment of migraine and headache requires collaboration between the doctor and patient; often the treatment goes beyond simple relief of symptoms because, during this collaboration, the patient frequently goes through a development and even the doctor does, too. The greatness of illness lies in its gift of creating the bases for healthy, selfless bonds between human beings.

As far as concerns *Ferrum-Quarz*, I recommend that you pay attention to your doctor's prescription, because often this is for capsules, while tablets are much less concentrated than the capsules and, therefore, reduce the possibility of healing considerably. The pills should be swallowed with water; in fact, in contrast to many other anthroposophic remedies, they should not be dissolved in the mouth.

Some practical advice
A useful remedy for providing relief from a headache is *Belladonna planta tota D4 drops*, 10 drops to be taken frequently – even every half hour – until the symptoms abate.
The effect of this remedy can be enhanced by *Chamomilla radix, ethanol decoctum D3 drops*, 10 drops, alternating the two remedies every half hour. It is worth being sure that the attack has been brought under control before reducing the dose.
Belladonna/Chamomilla globules, 5 globules every half hour; this contains the two remedies together in an alcohol-free formulation and is, therefore, ideal for children and adolescents and excellent for catamenial headache (headaches occurring during the menstrual cycle).
One very simple remedy is a *hot hand-bath*: submerge the hands up to the wrists in hot water; this is particularly useful for hangovers or headaches occurring during a diet, which develop as a sign of liberation from toxins.
Another remedy is a *cold footbath*. During an attack of headache, particularly when the head feels hot, put the feet into a bowl of cold water for a short time (from a few seconds to one or two minutes). The decongestant effect on the brain will be greater if

not only the feet, but also the legs from the knees downwards are put in cold water.

Coffee abstinence can cause a characteristic type of headache: in this case both cold footbaths and *Coffea D30 drops*, 7 drops in the morning are useful. These drops are also an excellent remedy in the case of insomnia due to an overflow of ideas, exactly as happens when someone drinks too much coffee. *Caffeine* can cause headache in people who do not tolerate this substance, associated in general with chocolate and tea, which contain theobromine and theophylline.

Nux vomica D6 drops, 10 drops every two or three hours; this is an excellent remedy for the hangover headache following too much alcohol the night before. With regards to migraine, the dangerous substance in alcoholic drinks, such as red wine, is tyramine, which is also found in cabbage and potatoes.

Bryonia D6 drops, 10 drops every two or three hours. This remedy is very useful in headaches extending from the forehead to the nape of the neck, making the head feel as if it is going to burst. This type of headache is worsened by movement, the person often has a dry mouth and constipation and is very irritable, flying into a rage over absolutely nothing.

Bloating and flatulence: wind imprisoned by the metabolism

"*According to the Pythagoreans, the flatulence after eating beans is due to dead spirits who inhabit these pulses and that, having entered the body, torment the people who have eaten them: in the day time with wind and during the night with nightmares. A nightmare is like a wind that is not expelled, circulating internally, rattling the shutters that protect the sleeping soul*" (Guido Ceronetti, Il silenzio del corpo, Adelphi, Milan 1979).

The technical term for bloating is *aerophagy*, which literally means "eating air". In reality, it is completely normal for air to be taken in with food and there is always a certain amount of air in the stomach, which is indispensable for the correct physiological function of this organ. It is commonly thought that when the abdomen is bloated or the person "feels a weight on the stomach" that he has swallowed too much air. Eating too quickly and drinking fizzy drinks are considered culprits. I believe that this point of view is too superficial, because it does not explain why so many people who eat fast and drink fizzy drinks do not suffer from bloating.

Meteorism, or flatulence, means the presence of air in the intestines, and is considered an expression of abnormal fermentation. Anthroposophic medicine explains that air is the physical substrate of the astral body, our emotional body; thus, every problem that concerns air also affects, to a variable extent, the astrality of the person as a whole. There is not a local disease or a local problem; the air in the abdomen is always the same, even if is manifested in two different areas of the body.

Obviously, some types of behaviour, such as eating fast, are both psychological factors (although we say soul factors) and promoters of changes to the air body within us. The treatment and prevention of aerophagy not only involve external habits, but also the whole person. Sometimes, when considering the clinical history of a patient, we can reach the conclusion that the tendency to flatulence is an expression of a shock, of an emotional trauma that has not been overcome; in these cases the treatment should take into account the personal history and find a way to heal and salve a wound to the soul. I remember having learnt from one of my patients that art therapy prescribed for other reasons corrected flatulence that had been the consequence of shock in the distant past, indications of which could also be seen in the patient's water colours.

The advice to chew thoroughly, if it is not just to be an empty catchphrase, must be accompanied by an examination of the factors that have led to an acceleration of our rhythms. In the end, if we manage to correct the mistaken habits and behaviours, we will be grateful to our aerophagy because it drove us to improve our quality of life.

Besides trying to chew thoroughly and avoiding fizzy drinks, the classical advice for bloating and flatulence is to decrease the intake of fruit and vegetables, because these ferment in the stomach or intestines and produce gas. I do not agree with this advice, because it is important for a person's general health to eat fruit and vegetables.

What should perhaps be done is to try to improve the digestibility of the fruit and vegetables, for example, by not eating fruit at the end of a substantial meal, but rather in the morning when the body's digestive capacity is at its peak, or away from main meals. Another way of improving the digestibility of fruit is to cook it, and limit the intake of prunes and raisins.

As far as concerns vegetables, the first useful piece of advice for those who tend to suffer from flatulence is to avoid mixing cooked and raw vegetables in the same meal. Raw vegetables cause less fermentation than cooked vegetable and go well with protein-based foods (main courses).

Cooked vegetables, although being less well tolerated by individuals susceptible to flatulence, combine well with cereal-based foods (pasta/rice dishes).

In summary:
1) mixing cooked and raw vegetables in the same meal causes flatulence in susceptible individuals;
2) raw vegetables are better tolerated than cooked ones in susceptible individuals because raw vegetables cause less fermentation;
3) from the perspective of digestive capacity, raw vegetables combine better with protein-based food; the classic meal of beefsteak and salad causes little flatulence even in susceptible subjects;
4) cooked vegetables, which are intrinsically more likely to cause flatulence, go well with cereals; for example, rice with pumpkin or radicchio (Italian chicory).

We all know that pulses provoke flatulence, promoting the formation of air as is well described in the quotation regarding the Pythagoreans at the beginning of this chapter. The strategy is not to eliminate them from the diet, but to cook them very well with spices and vegetables, which promote the digestion, and, above all, to avoid associating them with other pulses or protein-based foods, in particular those consisting of animal proteins.

Artificial sweeteners, such as sorbitol and mannitol, present in sugar-free dietary products, sweets and chewing-gum, promote the formation of gases, tricking the perceptive function of the digestion into believing that it is recognizing a sugar which actually is not present.

We should avoid food with a high content of fats, particularly saturated fats such as those in fried food, fatty meat, creamy sauces, rich condiments, whipped cream and industrial ice-creams which contain a lot of air. Lying down after a rich meal, laziness and physical inactivity promote the imprisonment of air within us.

Anthroposophic medicine tackles this problem with the measures described above, but also by trying to rebalance the astrality and the consequences that it has on our digestive system. Flatulence often also requires a personalised remedy that works on renal activity, since the kidney is a major organ involved in our astrality and emotions.

For example, vegetal charcoal, in the form of *Carbo Betulae*, birch charcoal, is actually an important remedy for kidney function, which helps to reduce and eliminate flatulence.

In brief, the strategies to prevent bloating and flatulence include:
– eating meals regularly, three times a day;
– avoiding tobacco smoke;
– eating in a quiet, relaxing place;
– eating fruit away from mealtimes;
– drinking away from mealtimes, at least six times a day, avoiding cold drinks;
– avoiding fizzy drinks and drinks rich in colorants;
– avoiding harmful or overly artificial foods;
– eliminating or reducing substances known by experience to cause the formation of wind;
– taking a personally prescribed, anthroposophic maintenance remedy which balances and harmonises our soul, our astral body.

Abdominal pain

This is a very important, delicate subject: in fact abdominal pain almost always requires the input of a doctor, whose diagnosis is indispensable. Here I am referring above all to *acute abdominal pain,* which often causes the patient not only intense suffering but also serious concern and necessitates a doctor's very swift interpretation and decisions, because in some cases, modest symptoms can hide more severe situations.
Chronic abdominal pain is a fairly frequent phenomenon; although not having the dramatic connotations and urgency of acute pain, it is often the source of severe limitations to the patient's social, occupational and, sometimes, emotional life. The search for the causes and the pathway towards the diagnosis are often very difficult and anthroposophic medicine can be of great help precisely because of its way of extending diagnostic and therapeutic horizons; in fact, it tends to take into consideration broader features and is not limited only to the "local" aspect of the symptoms.
However, the principle that abdominal pain is a challenging test of a doctor's diagnostic abilities holds true, because there are a huge number of conditions that can cause abdominal pain, the origin of the pain is very complex and the symptoms are often deceptive. These are the reasons why you should consult a doctor, rather, why you should consult a good doctor, in the case of abdominal pain and here there are no distinctions between schools or currents of thought (precisely for this reason, a person wanting to practice anthroposophic medicine must be a registered doctor!). For example, children with throat angina[49], even severe, do not have pain when swallowing, but very often the only symptom is a bothersome abdominal ache[50].

---

[49] *Angina* (from the Latin *angere,* "constrict"): this is a process producing a narrowing of the throat and, in general, the oropharynx (sore throat).
[50] This example highlights once again the relationship between the abdomen and the throat (between the metabolic system and disorders of the head) already described in the chapter on sore throat.

Part II. Illnesses and remedies

There are highly respected therapists who practice their discipline with passion and skill, but before consulting them, it is essential that the precise diagnosis is made. An osteopath, a physiotherapist, or a naturopath can do much to help in cases in which the abdominal pain is related to external factors, such as an irritated nerve due to the misalignment of spinal vertebrae, but these professionals cannot investigate whether there is a metastatic focus of cancer in the site of the pain or whether the gall bladder is not functioning correctly.

I make an appeal here against self-diagnosis and practices that could lose time or, worse, relieve symptoms that are diagnostically valuable. Considering acute abdominal pain, how many times have we seen an inflamed appendix, "masked" by self-prescribed treatments, even "natural" ones, or by antispasmodic drugs and analgesics, reach the stage of transformation into peritonitis?

A misunderstood acute abdomen can be life-threatening.

A patient can help the doctor greatly by noting and describing the features of his pain: the site, its characteristics (cramp-like, stabbing, stinging – that is, causing a burning sensation – etc.), how long it lasts, its rhythm (continuous, occasional, violent, intermittent, dull, etc.) and the factors that trigger it or that relieve it (eating food, passing a motion, urinating, posture, that is, the position that the patient takes to lessen the pain or because he is forced by the pain). Furthermore, any associated symptoms should not be neglected, even though these may be relieved or absent at the time of the doctor's examination: such symptoms include fever, vomiting, diarrhoea, jaundice (yellowish-brown colour of the skin), blood in the urine or faeces, very dark or black, sticky stool (a sign of bleeding in the stomach), transient loss of balance or collapse.

With regards to the diagnosis, the intensity of the pain is often very deceptive; in fact, apart from a few specific disorders such as renal and biliary colic or perforated ulcer, in many cases the perception of the pain is subjective and can vary greatly from one person to another.

It is interesting to appreciate that once the challenge of the diag-

Abdominal pain

nosis has been overcome successfully, both anthroposophic medicine and homeopathic medicine value precisely this subjectivity: the individual symptoms becomes extremely important for prescribing one remedy rather than another. Having made these introductory comments, let us now give some brief indications on specific subjects.

Biliary colic
Patients with biliary colic have really intense and sudden pain localised in the right epigastrium[51] which tends to radiate to the shoulder, the subscapular region and to the epigastrium[52]. These last two sites are very important for determining the cause of the pain. The onset of biliary colic is usually preceded by a large meal rich in fats. The pain is accompanied by nausea and almost always also by vomiting, which expels first the food eaten and then the bile juices.
The cause of the colic is the presence of one or more stones in the *gallbladder*, a sac which, between meals, collects the secretions from the liver, that is bile, which is excreted into the intestines during digestion through a small passage called the *common bile duct*. Colic is the result of attempts to expel a stone from the gallbladder.
Sometimes the stone is not formed in the gallbladder but in the *biliary tract*, and the attempts to expel the stone start from here. Colic is caused by the violent, spasmodic contractions of the walls of the ducts that the stone is passing through. However, the contractions tend to extend rapidly to other areas not directly involved by the irritant stimulus, so that other organs and functions should also be kept under observation. We can use some remedies while waiting for the doctor, who will make the diagnosis and decide the treatment.

---

[51] *Right epigastrium*: the region of the abdomen under the arch formed by the last ribs on the right; this region contains the right lobe of the liver, the gallbladder, the right kidney, the first curve of the duodenum and the bend between the ascending colon and the transverse colon (*right colonic flexure*).
[52] *Epigastrium*: the region corresponding to the upper area of the abdomen.

Part II. Illnesses and remedies

Belladonna planta tota D4 drops: 10 drops in water every half hour or even every fifteen minutes; this is an antispasmodic which relieves symptoms without causing problems. It can be combined with another remedy, *Oxalis folium D3 drops*: use 10 drops and alternate with *Belladonna* every 15-30 minutes; in the initial stages, the two remedies can even be given together, in a small amount of water or pouring the drops directly onto the tongue.

A decent, easy-to-use remedy is *Belladonna/Chamomilla globules*. In order to strengthen the treatment, globules of *Chelidonium/Colocinthis* can be added; these globules are formed of two remedies specific for the gallbladder, biliary dyskinesia[53] and spasms. Alternate 5-7 globules of the two remedies every 15-30 minutes, dissolving them in the mouth. When the pain has been stably relieved, reduce the frequency to every hour and do not suspend treatment abruptly, because this could lead to a recurrence of the painful crises.

Another good help is *Oxalis folium 10% ointment* to massage locally. Apply the cream, then a piece of wool and then carefully place a hot water bottle on the woollen cloth. This should only be used if the patient does not have a fever.

Another very useful remedy, again in the absence of a fever, is a compress made with a *tea of Achillea millefolium (yarrow)*. Pour a tablespoon of *yarrow* into half a litre of boiling water, cover the vessel and leave to steep for ten minutes and filter; dip a piece of wool into the tea and, after having squeezed it, apply it locally, cover with a small towel and place a hot water bottle on top to maintain the warmth.

Fever is an important symptom of abdominal disorders and should make us consult a doctor urgently. Once the doctor has made the diagnosis, the same remedies described above can be given with good effect by injection (for example *Belladonna D4 vial, Oxalis Rh D3 vial*), administered subcutaneously along the

---

[53] *Biliary dyskinesia*: an abnormality in the neurovegetative coordination of the smooth muscle of the gallbladder; in practice, this is an alteration in the balanced rhythm of contractions of the gallbladder which enable adequate secretion of bile after meals.

Abdominal pain

pathway of the pain in well-known pain points, such as the cystic point, which is also a diagnostic point for colic. This treatment is often extraordinarily effective in providing immediate relief.

The application of *cups over the liver* is another very effective remedy; the doctor or better still the anthroposophic nurse[54] can apply these or show the patient how to use them. These are glass cups in which a vacuum is created by a flame. Applied to the skin, the effect of the vacuum is to draw blood to the surface: this increases local warmth, helping to reduce spasms and congestion of the area.

An archetypal remedy for the gallbladder

Anthroposophic medicine obtains interesting results in the treatment and prevention of colic using a very important background remedy which must be prescribed by a doctor and taken for a long time. This remedy is *Chelidonium/Curcuma drops*: the dose is from 10 to 15 drops after the three daily meals in half a glass of warm water or in an tea of yarrow. This is one of the "archetypal remedies" of anthroposophic medicine created by the pharmaceutical genius of Rudolf Steiner, which we mentioned when discussing *Cardiodoron* in the chapter on aerophagy and flatulence. It is unlikely that surgery will be needed if this remedy is used well. I am, of course, against self-prescription because initially this treatment can worsen symptoms because of its effect of stimulating contraction of the gallbladder; this remedy must be welcomed by the body, which means working on the sympathetic forces present in metabolic functions.

---

[54] Anthroposophic medicine strongly values numerous professionals, in particular *nurses*, who carry out precious and indispensable work in clinics and can administer a range of treatments, including yarrow compresses and vacuum cups. Although defending the prerogative of the doctor in making a clinical diagnosis, I would like to highlight that the opinion of the nurse is very much taken into consideration in anthroposophic clinics also with regards to the choice of treatment, because sometimes external treatment and anthroposophic plant remedies are more effective than subcutaneous injections. Anthroposophic medicine was founded and can develop in a healthy community, and for this reason we elderly doctors, who have had to work alone in our surgeries, look to the future with optimism.

Part II. Illnesses and remedies

Renal colic

Renal colic is a particularly painful crisis due to the passage of a stone through the *ureter,* the long, narrow tube connecting the kidney to the bladder. Pain can be present towards the back in the flank region and towards the front in the abdomen on the side of the affected kidney. The pain can also radiate to the genitals and thighs. While waiting for the doctor, the advice is bed rest, a hot water bottle over the kidney and natural antispasmodics, as for biliary colic: *Belladonna D4 drops* and *Oxalis D3*, alternating 10 drops of the two remedies every 15-30 minutes; *Belladonna/Chamomilla*, 10 globules every half hour, may also be useful. Likewise, *Belladonna comp. suppositories*, one suppository every 4-6 hours, are also useful for pain relief. Another effective remedy is *Oxalis 10% ointment* applied over the kidney and along the pathway of the pain, that is, between the ureter and iliac fossa on the affected side. Once applied, the ointment is covered with a woollen cloth before holding a hot water bottle to the affected part. A specific, symptomatic remedy for colic is *Berberis decoctum (cortex) D3 drops*, 10 drops every half hour alternated with *Belladonna D4*. The doctor will use the same antispasmodic remedies, but in vial form, injecting it along the pain pathway and at certain points specific for kidney pain, in the same way as for biliary colic. If the stone does not move or becomes lodged, traditional analgesics could become necessary.

The application of *vacuum cups* along the pain pathway is also useful, although less effective than in biliary colic. *As far as concerns drinking,* you should wait for the doctor or until the phase of acute colicky pain has passed; in fact, drinking could risk intensifying the pain because it increases the pressure on, and swelling of, the affected kidney. Only when the pain has lifted does it become useful to drink large amounts of water with a low mineral content.

Right-sided renal colic can generally be distinguished from biliary colic because the pain from renal colic tends to localise or at least to radiate to the right iliac fossa[55]; furthermore, in renal colic

---

[55] *Right iliac fossa:* the right, lower part of the abdomen.

there tends to be a characteristic restlessness and agitation which can help the diagnosis and confirms the astral nature (emotional sphere) of renal physiology.

An archetypal remedy for kidney stones
The anthroposophic remedy *Lapis Cancri/Acidum silicicum naturale D15 tablets* is a formidable strategy for preventing the formation of new kidney stones once the ones causing the acute attack have been expelled; it also has an anti-inflammatory effect and can control the growth of existing stones. It can be used for prophylactic purposes in subjects who have clinical or laboratory indicators of a predisposition to the development of stones, such as the continuous presence of calcium oxalate crystals in the urine. This remedy, designed by Steiner, stems from little river crabs which are able to "save" calcium, putting it apart, before moulting, in the form of tiny stones in the stomach (gastroliths); subsequently these stones are dissolved and the calcium that was saved is used in the new shell. It is this great ecological wisdom, this balance, of the river crab, which is the therapeutic gesture that inspired the formulation of the remedy, to which silica is added: this latter is a powerful anti-inflammatory agent and a re-balancer, nowadays one would say *modulator,* of the immune system.

Acute appendicitis
The most common cause of acute abdominal pain in the right iliac fossa is *acute appendicitis.* Often preceded by general malaise and disorders of apparently gastric origin (pain in the epigastrium, nausea and/or vomiting), acute appendicitis is manifested by a persistent pain, often localised in the epigastrium in the area around the navel and, of course, in the right lower quadrant of the abdomen; the pain can irradiate, depending on the anatomical position of the appendix, to the thigh (characteristically, there is a feeling of the leg "pulling"), to the pelvis, to the navel, etc. The simultaneous presence of sudden constipation is very common. There is a characteristic tenderness in the right iliac fossa which becomes much more painful when the palpating hand is

removed abruptly from the abdomen (Blumberg's sign). The inflamed appendix can perforate, causing peritonitis or the formation of an appendix abscess.

For this reason, *a patient with pain in the lower right part of the abdomen and around the navel should contact his doctor urgently or go to hospital, particularly if he has a fever over 38°C and if the patient is between 9 and 16 years old.*

While waiting for the doctor it is useful to measure the *rectal temperature* and the *axillary temperature,* after having carefully dried away any sweat from the armpit, and compare the two. A clear difference of more than half a degree centigrade (a physiological difference) is a sign of intestinal inflammation. In this case local *applications of ice* are appropriate and it is advisable not to eat or drink[56]. Laxatives and enemas are absolutely forbidden. In order to avoid complicating the diagnosis for the doctor, who must decide whether to start a treatment or organize an immediate admission to hospital, I recommend minimising or excluding the use of the anthroposophic antispasmodic remedies described for biliary colic, and even more so, synthetic antiaspasmodic drugs.

In my experience, one of the most common causes of a worsening appendicitis in youngsters is dietary errors and, I'm afraid I have to say it, *chocolate, in all its "versions", is the number one culprit.* It is known that holidays are the period in which there is a peak in the onset of acute appendicitis. Another risk factor is *poor quality fats,* in particular fried fats and "strange" creams. *Fried potatoes* in any form, but particularly crisps, together with all the types of food stuffed with preservatives, such as the numerous snacks which often combine frying with cocoa powder, are enemy number two of the appendix, because they cause intestinal inflammation.

The predisposition to appendix disorders does, however, stem

---

[56] I apologise to the readers for the obviousness of some indications, such as *"fast during an abdominal illness"*, but I believe it is better to be slightly boring than leave a patient to make dangerous errors and risk worsening his condition. Nowadays, despite the barrage of information, there is a lack of the most elementary knowledge of traditional family medicine that all doctors agree on.

Abdominal pain

from an excess of animal proteins, especially meat, which alter the intestinal bacterial flora and slow the transit of material through the bowel, forcing the appendix to work without interruption in an unbalanced environment. This happens in the second septennium (from 7 to 14 years) in which the appendix becomes the school where white blood cells learn the essential information for our defences and for the future of our immune system. Precisely in this age period, our children become more autonomous and just "get" the food suggested by advertising and by greed, increasing the risk of harming the appendix, which is the 'schoolmistress' of the intestinal immune system and the most important organ of our defences in that stage of life. In my opinion, the prevention of disorders of the appendix is, therefore, based particularly on the type of diet. I can state that among the youngsters I have cared for, the few who have had to undergo an appendicectomy were almost always "consumers" of chocolate and chips.

Another factor predisposing to damage to the appendix is *tonsillectomy in the first septennium,* which fortunately is now very rarely performed because it has been understood how important it is for the immune system to have fully functioning, in sequential order, *the three great schools for training white blood cells*:

0-1   First year of life: maternal milk

0-7   First septennium: tonsils and adenoids

7-14   Second septennium: appendix vermiformis

Abdominal colic

This is a painful crisis, sometimes very violent, localised to the abdomen. People who suffer from this problem have easily irritated intestines (irritable bowel syndrome) or constipation. Although it is a chronic condition, there may be acute painful crises with or without diarrhoea. A history of chronic bowel disease can, however, be reassuring, allowing the use of the already described antispasmodics, such as *Belladonna/Chamomilla*, 5 globules every half hour, a *hot water bottle* or *a chamomile compress* (see later);

once the pain has improved, these remedies should be gradually used less frequently.

One good remedy, specific for preventing crises but also excellent in the acute stage, is *Chamomilla/Nicotiana globules*: start with 5 globules every half hour and then, as the symptoms lessen, reduce to 10 globules every two hours and then 10 globules before the three meals until assessment by the doctor, who will decide further treatment.

Patients who have unexpected abdominal colic must be evaluated by a doctor urgently, in order to exclude very serious problems such as appendicitis, stones, pancreatitis, ulcers, diverticulitis, or intestinal obstruction. Changes must be made to the diet to prevent further attacks of abdominal colic: if the individual is constipated, he must eat fibre-rich food (fruit, pulses, cooked green and bitter vegetables, well-cooked biodynamic wholemeal cereals); if, on the other hand, he has diarrhoea, the advice given in the specific chapter on this subject should be followed.

Windy colic in the baby

Babies inevitably produce gas in the intestines, this being part of their need to harmonise with the new food they are introducing as well as dealing with the dietary habits and emotional life of their mother and family.

The first rule is undoubtedly to establish a *good rhythm for the feeds*. After an initial harmonisation and stimulation of lactation, a feed should be given about every four hours, trying to reach a slightly longer interval in the night. I am against feeding on demand for the simple reason that adding fresh milk to semi-digested milk in the stomach can cause fermentation and, therefore, *meteorism*[57]. We need to listen to the needs of babies, taking time, lulling them and giving them a *tea of fennel seeds* (biological or better still biodynamic): put half a teaspoon of the seeds into a napkin and crush them lightly with a meat tenderiser be-

---

[57] Remember that meteorism is a swelling of the abdomen due to gas in the gastrointestinal tract, usually caused by fermentation of food.

Abdominal pain

fore adding them to a quarter of a litre of boiling water; filter after ten minutes.

A few teaspoons of the tea can be given before every feed in order to prevent the baby developing too much wind. With regards to the warmth body, it should be remembered that this is not yet balanced in an infant. If a baby has cold hands and feet, he needs to be warmed, which can be done, with prudence, by putting a hot water bottle in the cot; do not forget the importance of a cotton or linen bonnet. True windy colic is characterized by uncontrollable crying which starts suddenly in a moment of apparent well-being; it often occurs in the evening and can last up to several hours.

The colic is caused by slowed transit through the intestines, which distends the intestinal walls because of excess formation of gas. Some babies are particularly sensitive to intestinal stimuli.

Another cause of windy colic is that the mother's diet contains too much fresh milk, eggs or pulses, or the mother has an intolerance of cow's milk. In this case the mother must alter her diet to eliminate milk and dairy products. A good remedy for meteorism is to massage the baby's abdomen above and around the navel with *Cuprum 0.4% ointment*. This massage should be done a couple of times a day, always in a clockwise (looking at the child) direction and possibly in the hours preceding a potential colic attack: since this is typically the evening, massage the baby around four o'clock in the afternoon.

Chamomilla D6 drops: these are used if the baby, usually peaceful, starts screaming and kicking, and can only be calmed by being taken for a walk or, above all, a car ride. The dose is 5 drops in the fennel tea at room temperature before every feed.

Chamomilla Cupro culta, radix Rh D3 drops: this is a very useful and effective remedy in more severe attacks. In this case, too, the dose is 5 drops in the fennel tea given before every feed.

Magnesit D3 trituration: while the child screams and kicks, he also sweats. This remedy is effective in breastfed babies, with greenish, frothy faeces, particularly when the baby is opening his bowels frequently. The colic makes the baby bend his legs upwards towards the chest. Dissolve a small pinch of the powder in the fennel tea and give before every feed.

During the colic attacks, give the recommended remedies, dissolving them in a spoonful of tea, as often as every one or two hours.

A chamomile compress is also excellent to prevent attacks.

Chamomile compresses for the abdominal area

Chamomile compresses are widely used by anthroposophic doctors for abdominal disorders; in fact, they help with gastrointestinal disorders, recurrent vomiting, colic, windy colic in babies, abdominal pain and cramps. They should be avoided in cases of pain in the lower part of the abdomen, because the warmth can be harmful in the case of inflammation of the appendix.

The compress is prepared by submerging a small terry towel, rolled up on itself, into a hot chamomile tea. The tea is made by pouring a tablespoon of chamomile flowers into a litre of boiling water, covering the recipient well and filtering after at least ten minutes.

Having checked that the temperature is tolerable, particularly if the patient is a baby, apply the towel to the painful area and cover it with a larger woollen cloth. A hot water bottle can be added to increase the efficacy of the compress. Keep in place for about 15 minutes, possibly repeating the treatment after one or two hours.

Diarrhoea

In the previous chapter we tried to give some information useful for orienting oneself in the complex situation of painful abdominal disorders. In this chapter we want to provide some brief indications on how to tackle diarrhoea[58], a disorder characterized by expulsion of faeces, of a greater volume, more liquid and at a higher frequency than normal, often accompanied by abdominal pain, fever and vomiting. The acute form is usually due to having eaten food containing toxins, to intestinal infections or to altered intestinal transit; this form almost always heals spontaneously.

Diarrhoea can lead to a loss of fluids and electrolytes (potassium, sodium, chloride, magnesium, etc.) with consequent *dehydration* and *collapse*. Furthermore, metabolic acidosis may develop as a result of the loss of bicarbonates, hypotonia and weakness because of the decrease in potassium (hypokalaemia) and spasms because of a drop in magnesium. The presence of blood in the faeces and continuous abdominal pain are signs that should raise alarm.

In the case in which the symptoms are particularly pronounced and dangerous, especially in children and in the elderly, the patient should be seen by a doctor or go to the Accident and Emergency department in order that the fluid-electrolyte balance can be restored quickly.

The same holds true in the case of diarrhoea lasting more than two weeks: this requires a diagnosis because it could be related to an important food intolerance, inflammatory bowel disease, serious infection (typhus, cholera) or cancer of the colon.

---

[58] We have no embarrassment in using the term *diarrhoea* which is correct, since it is derived from the Greek *dia* ("through") and *rein* ("flow"). Use of the word *dysentery*, a technical medical term for specific disorders in which the diarrhoea presents with few stools containing mucus and/or blood, is certainly not as elegant and refined as many people believe.

Semiliquid diet in acute diarrhoea

Acute diarrhoea in babies and children should be treated with a diet based exclusively on teas, without added sugar, such as *very bland tea,* a *tea of chamomile*, a pre-prepared *tea of dried or fresh blueberries*. To prepare the blueberries tea, put five teaspoons of berries in half a litre of cold water and then boil for five minutes, filter and drink three cups a day. After one day of drinking only teas, the patient can start eating again, as indicated below in the section on a semiliquid diet.

Infants, in particular, should be given rice pudding (simply use white rice cooked for a long time in a generous amount of water), grated apple with lemon juice, a mash of boiled carrots, which is prepared by simmering 500 grams of carrots in a litre of water with a little salt for two hours. The carrots must be biodynamic or biological, because those grown in land that has been fertilised with chemicals may have a high content of nitrates, which inflame the mucosa.

As I have already stated, it is really important that biodynamic foods are used for babies and children.

A *semiliquid diet* based on substances rich in magnesium and potassium is an important measure in acute diarrhoea. Let us have a look at such a diet. Generous amounts of chamomile tea or tea with lemon should be drunk. Sugar-free blueberry juice with added fresh lemon juice or a drink of blended carrot and apple is also allowed. The diet should consist of *food with minimal waste residues*. The base of the diet is polished rice with its rice water, carrot mash, grated apple, and biological bananas mashed with lemon. To begin with, condiments such as oil and sugar, and also bread, should be avoided. Milk and all protein foods are forbidden until a balance is restored. At this point slices of toast, not of wholemeal bread, can be introduced, followed by white yoghurt at room temperature.

It is important to understand that biodynamic wholemeal bread, although very healthy, is rich in roughage and is not, therefore, appropriate during the recovery from diarrhoea. White rice is the most suitable cereal, whereas the wonderful oatmeal, so rich in nutritional value, stimulates peristalsis (intestinal contractions) too much.

Traditional food can then be introduced into the diet, but no more than one new type of food, which should be easily digestible, per meal. So, spaghetti with a drop of olive oil rather than "spaghetti Bolognese". Grilled meat rather than cutlets or meat cooked with butter. There is no point in being in a hurry after a major bout of diarrhoea, you must give time for the irritated mucosa and intestinal bacterial flora to recover.

In any case, dietary measures help to limit the damage caused by the losses also in the cases of diarrhoea requiring intervention from the doctor. Let us turn now to some of the basic remedies.

Basic remedies

Chamomilla radix D3 drops: these drops are important when the contractions of the intestines are too strong and are extremely useful in teething babies and small children. The dose is 10 drops every two hours in the adult and from 3 to 7 drops in children.

Belladonna/Chamomilla globules: this is an excellent remedy for forms of diarrhoea with fever caused by viral infection, typical of the change of season in the autumn and spring. The dose is from 3 to 7 globules even as often as every half hour in the case of intestinal cramps and a temperature that is tending to rise. This remedy is a natural spasmolytic also useful for adults. In some children (the irritable, temperamental, "chamomile type" child of homeopathy) the remedy can induce sleepiness, which is often welcomed by the parents, exhausted by the rebellious nature of their little offspring. These globules do not contain lactose, but are based on saccharose and can, therefore, be used in subjects with lactose intolerance.

Geum urbanum Rh D3 drops: these drops are useful for diarrhoea caused by poor digestion and abdominal bloating and for summer diarrhoea with characteristically acrid stools, often due to overeating or eating foods that are too "wintery". This is a typical non-alcoholic paediatric remedy. The dose is from 3 to 7 drops every one or two hours in a little water or directly in the mouth. Together with the diet described, it can prevent or cure an acute gastroenteritis. It is, therefore, one of those remedies typical of anthroposophic medicine which is a profound help, starting from the principle of wanting to support the body's functions, in this case lightening the load on the weakened activity of the "I" in metabolism. Indeed, the warmth body cannot stay in equilibrium and a fever appears. This remedy is useful in acute febrile diarrhoea because it helps to prevent recurrences when the patient starts to eat food again.

Levico D3 drops: this typically anthroposophic remedy originates from the precious mineral water of Levico[59], a so-called "strong water", a valuable, natural alchemy of arsenic, copper, iron, zinc and many other metals and oligo-elements. This is a way of giving arsenic, vitalised not only by potentisation, as in the typical homeopathic remedy for diarrhoea, but also by the miraculous life arising from the meeting between heaven and earth in the water that runs through the mountains. This is a remedy that is capable of supporting and harmonising the astral body in its task of creating secretions. It is useful in cases of weakness if the stools are very liquid and voided violently. The dose is 10 drops every two hours in adults and from 3 to 7 drops in children. Alternated every hour, at the usual doses, with *Geum urbanum Rh D3*, it is effective in the treatment of *summer diarrhoea*.

Stibium m.p. D6 trituration: this is a remedy that acts deeply and should, therefore, be prescribed by a doctor; it is based on antimony, an element that provides profound support to the metabolic sphere and digestion, starting from the blood. We mention

---

[59] The springs of Levico Vetriolo and Roncegno, close to Trento (Italy), were already known from the late Mediaeval period. In his first course for doctors, in 1920, Steiner stated that "This water seems to have been prepared by some kindly spirit and certain forces can be found there in nature, which play a fundamental role in the human organism. In these thermal waters, the forces of both copper and iron are found in admirably balanced proportions, which are given a broader base by traces of arsenic". Levico water is at the centre of the therapeutic activities of the Raphael Health Centre at Roncegno (Italy), where patients are treated with anthroposophic medicine.

it to help understand the reasons why a doctor prescribes a remedy that acts on the metabolic man, where the shaping forces (which create and maintain form) give way to the metabolism and the substance tends to escape from the control of the organization of "I": it is, therefore, useful in the various types of bleeding, in diarrhoea, particularly if haemorrhagic, and in eczemas. For example, it plays an important role in ulcers of the stomach and duodenum, but also in severe chronic inflammatory bowel diseases, such as ulcerative colitis and Crohn's disease.

Nux vomica D4 dilution: this is a useful remedy for acute diarrhoea accompanied by frequent vomiting, often related to the presence of food toxins that the body tries to eliminate. The dose is from 7 to 10 drops every ten minutes, diluted in a teaspoon of cool tea, thus avoiding too much liquid, which could stimulate more vomiting. Once the acute phase has been overcome, reduce the frequency of administration but continue the diet for at least three days.

Veratrum album ethanol decoctum D4 dilution: this is useful in acute diarrhoea with debilitation, copious cold sweats, a feeling of cold throughout the body and strong pain before evacuating the bowels followed by a lack of strength. For children use *Levico D3* first and in more severe cases alternate the two remedies every one or two hours. This alternation of the two remedies is particularly useful in summer diarrhoea with fermentation and sour-smelling stool.

Bolus alba comp. N powder: this is useful for harmonising the digestive processes in the case of diarrhoea with marked peristalsis and widespread inflammation of the gastrointestinal tract. This remedy is based on white clay (kaolin), but also contains arsenic (which is effective in the treatment of diarrhoea) in homeopathic doses. The dose is a teaspoon of the powder in a cup of warm water: take sips every one or two hours. As the symptoms improve, reduce the frequency of the treatment to three or four times a day and continue to obtain a more profound curative effect.

Lactic acid bacteria: are really useful in diarrhoea, particularly to restore the balance of the intestinal flora, these bacteria are indispensable, as everyone knows, in the case of diarrhoea occuring after the use of antibiotics, which alter this balance. You should use probiotic lactic acid bacteria cultures grown on a malt substrate, not a milk based one, because this could worsen the diarrhoea in the case of lactose intolerance. Being unfair to many other good products, I mention here *Rhamnoselle*, which acts specifically in the colon. The dose in the acute phase is three capsules a day, and then reduced to two and then one capsule a day: terrain treatments[60] and natural remedies are not usually stopped abruptly.

---

[60] In complementary medicine, terrain treatments mean specific remedies that are prescribed by a doctor on the basis of the patient's individual characteristics and that are aimed at improving the patient's reactivity and general well-being.

Traveller's diarrhoea and summer food poisoning

"Montezuma's revenge"
The most common problem for travellers is diarrhoea. Doctors are often consulted about this problem and some useful considerations are presented in the chapter on a change of air. Traveller's diarrhoea, popularly called "Montezuma's revenge"[61], an illness known for centuries, is due in most cases[62] to food and drinks contaminated by potentially virulent pathogenic micro-organisms which, by multiplying, alter the intestinal bacterial flora. The main symptom is the passage of three or more unformed stools a day. These diarrhoeal discharges are often accompanied by nausea, fever, cramps, abdominal pain and vomiting. Although this is not usually a serious disorder and resolves spontaneously within a few days, it faithfully obeys Murphy's law[63] and

---

[61] Montezuma II (1466-1520), Aztec emperor of Mexico who surrendered pacifically to Hernán Cortés, identifying him as the divine Quetzalcoatl, and who died following the rebellion triggered by the Mexicans against the Spanish invaders. Although the Spaniards prevailed over the natives, they were subsequently decimated by an epidemic caused by the infected, local water. Even nowadays, we still use the term "Montezuma's revenge" to refer to the infections frequently contracted by people who travel through some areas of Mexico and Latin America (but also the Middle East, Asia and Africa). The infection is transmitted through water from places without adequate purification. Although travellers may be careful not to drink local water, they often become infected by cleaning their teeth with this water or drinking beverages cooled with ice made from the local water or eating food prepared with this water. Montezuma had welcomed Cortés as a divinity but was humiliated by the Spaniards: it is still said nowadays that the water of his land wreaks his revenge on foreigners.

[62] Also called "the disease of the three 'Fs'": *flies, fingers, food*, referring to the methods of contamination.

[63] Murphy's law is the invention of an America humourist and has become the source of self-deprecating reflection for millions of adepts all over the world, including myself. The law goes something like this: "*If something can go wrong, it will*". Naturally, there are infinite variations of the theme, both in books published on aphorisms and in anecdotes recounted orally, but you can make your

ruins the trip, particularly if in tropical countries or in the summer holidays. For this reason, and I hope without shocking anyone, I teach my patients some principles of so-called *travel medicine*. The principles also apply to summer diarrhoea, caused by food poisoning due to the ingestion of bacteria contained in contaminated food.

Prevention
Primary prevention consists of avoiding some raw foods, such as seafood, meat, unwashed vegetables, milk and dairy products, which are often not preserved correctly, as well as some cooked foods such as puddings containing fresh cream or crême pâtissière, which should be kept in a refrigerator. However, above all, it is essential not to drink water or beverages that are not bottled. It must be remembered that the number one enemy is ice, which besides being made of water of unknown source, is regularly picked up by hands that are never sterile. Furthermore, as is well known, cold weakens the intestinal immune system, facilitating the growth of harmful bacteria.

In order to prevent and control changes in the intestinal bacterial flora caused by alterations in dietary habits during holidays in distant places, it is useful to take *"probiotics"* each day; the high concentration of lactic acid bacteria in these products block the growth of the undesirable bacteria in the intestines. These probiotics should be taken from the start of the trip and continued for at least seven to ten days, even if you return home within a week. If symptoms develop, the dose can be increased to three times a day. It is also important to follow the semiliquid diet described in the previous chapter.

In the case of persistent symptoms, with more severe diarrhoea (three or more bowel movements in eight hours) I advise trav-

own taking inspiration from daily life, in which this law invariably triumphs. Personally, since I am disorganized, I come up against it every day: whatever tactic I use to search for a particular sheet of paper among a pile, the one that I am looking for is always the last! So I have learned to go methodically through my notes, without trying any short-cuts which invariably worsen the situation.

ellers in the tropics to take a specific, selective antibiotic that acts in the intestines. My preference is *Rifaximin* (Xifaxan), which it is useful to carry with you. It does not have major, general effects on the body and has minimal interactions with other drugs. It can also be given to children. Of course I also advise drinking and taking an oral rehydration salt *containing potassium and magnesium,* which is always worth carrying with you together with the probiotics, because a hot climate and diarrhoea quickly deplete the body's stores of salts.

In cases of *summer diarrhoea* and *food poisoning* the same remedies as those described in the previous chapter can be used, provided it will be possible to obtain the suggested remedy.
I would like to remind you of three very interesting and useful remedies for food poisoning, noting that all the dietary advice given previously is valid in this situation, too. In fact, nowadays we easily commit dietary errors and often holidays and festivities are occasions for excesses which end up making ourselves and other people unhappy.
Pulsatilla D6 granules or *drops*: this is a remedy for the gastroenteritis that occurs in children and adults after having eaten fatty foods, too much ice-cream, fruit or different foods (onions, pork, fruit, ice-cream) or simply too much. There is diarrhoea, but also vomiting. The stools differ from each other as if they were "telling" a mystery tale: one green, one scrambled egg-like... The diagnosis is confirmed by the patina covering the tongue and the strong thirst which tells us of the need to "dilute and homogenise" the extraneous food that has penetrated us. The dose is 3 granules or 10 drops every two hours in adults and 2 granules or 5 drops every two hours in children.
Arsenicum album D6 or *D10 drops*: this is a suitable remedy for poisoning due to meat that has gone off, but also in my clinical experience, food poisoning from contaminated oysters. The attack occurs about 24 hours after eating the affected food and is sudden and violent, a bolt from the blue, especially if the vomiting and diarrhoea develop almost simultaneously and have an ex-

plosive nature; the patient has violent, burning pain in the abdomen which causes despair, intense agitation and, as the great homeopathic doctors say, fear of dying. The faeces are dark, bloody, smelly and scarce. The astral body is certainly provoked and will try desperately to free itself from the strong hold of the toxins that imprison it in the metabolism. The vomiting and diarrhoea, attempting to void the body from both the top and the bottom end, are its response, in a brilliant military strategy: "if there are too many enemies to tackle, a diversionary manoeuvre is necessary to decrease their number".

We are faced with a severe clinical picture, with incipient dehydration; nevertheless, let me tell you that if the situation is as described you should, indeed, call your doctor, but while waiting to see him, you can experience the extraordinary speed and strength of anthroposophic and homeopathic medicine, by taking 10 drops of this remedy every one or two hours.

The effect is sometimes so intense that, after a brief worsening for two or three hours, the patient recovers strength and does not open his bowels again for three or four days.

I have personally witnessed formidable results and was left admiring and enthusiastic.

Okoubaka D3 tablets: these tablets are a homeopathic remedy for food poisoning with diarrhoea caused by rotten food or food that has gone bad because it has been preserved incorrectly. If there is continuous nausea, vomiting and general malaise, dissolve one tablet in the mouth three or four times a day. This remedy is very suitable for children at the same doses and is also indicated for traveller's diarrhoea.

Constipation: holding nature within us

Chronic constipation is one of the most common disorders afflicting people in industrialised countries. It is considered "the mother of all illnesses of civilisation".
Regularly emptying the bowels is of great importance for health, not only because the intestines can be a source of toxins, but also because they are the site of the largest organ of the immune system and of the intestinal flora, which are of fundamental importance for the equilibrium of the whole body[64].
Constipation is a source of infinite psychophysical distress and is characterized by infrequent bowel movements because of slowed transit of the digestive waste through the intestines; this leads to scarce, hard stools, difficult or painful defecation, and abnormal and incomplete emptying of the sigmoid colon and rectum. The frequency of passing motions varies from person to person.
The treatment consists of removing the faecal pressure and re-establishing the habit of soft stools and painless transit. The proper, chronic form of constipation starts in infancy and is often related to bad lifestyle habits.
In 90-95% of children with constipation, no apparent organic cause is found. There may be a combination of factors related to a diet with a low fibre content and family characteristics. Psychosocial factors are often suggested to be involved, although most children with constipation have a normal development.
Chronic constipation can lead to progressive faecal retention, distension of the rectum and loss of sensory and motor function of the intestines. Constipation rarely has an organic cause.
The most frequent origin of constipation is certainly a diet of refined foods poor in fibre and inadequate fluid intake. Scarce

---

[64] With regards to the intestinal microflora, this plays a key role in the gastrointestinal ecosystem and is essential for normal, physiological development of the intestinal immune system, known as the GALT (gastrointestinal mucosa associated lymphoid tissue) which alone contains 40% of all the immune cells in the human body.

physical activity also contributes, as demonstrated by the frequent onset of constipation after prolonged bed rest. Unfortunately many synthetic drugs promote constipation; here I shall mention only antacids, antidepressants, anxiolytics, many antihypertensive drugs, for example beta-blockers, laxatives, muscle relaxants, analgesics and toxic metals (arsenic, lead, mercury).

Let me summarise the three groups of causes of the three types of constipation:

1) over-refined foods, lacking fibre, which do not, therefore, adequately stimulate the movements of the walls of the colon;

2) sedentary lifestyle and poor intestinal and abdominal muscle tone with a deficiency in the mechanisms of expelling the faeces;

3) alterations and disturbances of the reflex nervous mechanisms that automatically regulate the emptying of the bowel.

Once the causes of the constipation have been understood and eliminated, the intestine must be re-educated in order that it starts to function regularly again. This education is based on following the principles of a healthy diet, as we have repeatedly discussed in this book.

It is useful to increase the *fibre content in the diet* in order to increase the bulk of the stools, the frequency of evacuation and the speed of transit. In the presence of fibre, more bile is eliminated with the faeces and so the liver makes more; since it does this starting from cholesterol, this has the effect of reducing the concentration of cholesterol circulating in the bloodstream. We can all understand now how the control of cholesterol levels is one of the fundamental "rejuvenating factors" of a diet based on wholemeal cereals. By introducing or increasing the amount of biological or biodynamic wholemeal cereals in our diet, we are working to achieve a good "ecological" balance in our body, but we are also making a contribution to the health of mother Earth, made more fertile by healthy husbandry. Besides the classic wholemeal rice, I mention cereals that can be added to vegetable soups, in particular oatmeal which is delicate and produces a precious mucilage. Fruit and vegetables are indispensable, especially local products eaten in the correct period of ripeness.

Learning to chew thoroughly is of great importance, particularly in the case of food rich in fibres, such as wholemeal cereals, which, in order to be well tolerated, must be chewed adequately. Chewing not only helps mechanical transformation of food and its sufficient mixing with digestive enzymes, but it also allows the food to be tasted well, which is the first stage in the long and complex metamorphosis that is the most important aspect of the digestive process. Thorough chewing enables a better perception of the amount and components of food and determines the sense of satiety.

One of the important causes of overeating, typical of our times, is precisely that of eating food that is too refined and too easily assimilated, which does not require much chewing and which does not, therefore induce a sense of satiation.

Physical activity and walks are essential to activate our metabolism; constipation is a state of stasis, a slowing, and is treated with movement in its infinite forms. I advise exercise every day.

Laxatives

"The rule is: laxatives make constipation a chronic condition"
It is difficult to treat constipation with drugs, as demonstrated by the impressive number of laxative drugs on sale. Considering the intestine as an independent organ on which to act directly is yet another example of the principle of one-sidedness. Constipation should be tackled starting from the idea that the whole body participates in the intestinal process and that also our lifestyle takes part. In substance, the immense arsenal of treatments for constipation, whether synthetic or natural, is based on three different strategies.

The *first* strategy is to *"accelerate the transit"*. Generally speaking, the drugs that have this effect tend to irritate the mucosa of the large bowel[65], increasing the blood flow in the area; this stimu-

---

[65] Large bowel: the last part of the intestine that goes from the ileo-caecal valve to the anus. It includes the caecum, the vermiform appendix, the colon, the rectum and the anus. Its function is to reabsorb the fluids from within the intestine.

lates the muscles of the intestine to contract, causing those abdominal cramps that are well known to all users of laxatives and the violent expulsion of the contents of the intestine. Over time the intestine gets used to this irritation and the dose of the laxative must be progressively increased in order to obtain the desired effect.

The *second* strategy is based on irritation of nerves; the so-called *"dilators"* produce a dilatory irritation on the walls of the intestine, which reacts by expelling its contents. However, as time passes, the intestine becomes accustomed and the effect is decreased or lost.

The *third* strategy, of *"lubrication"*, is equally problematic. This has a purely mechanical effect that obviously weakens the autonomous activity of the intestine. *We can say that chronic constipation is the result of a process of weakening intestinal activity.*

The wisest thing to do which obeys the laws of life is to stop mistreating the poor intestine and start a process towards restoring adequate function which will require, like every change, a certain time and patience by the person who must undertake it.

The same philosophical patience that we use when learning a new sport, knowing that it will take us a certain time to learn it, must be applied to the management of constipation, without being carried away by a harmful desire to "be in a hurry".

A fundamental remedy that your doctor will prescribe is *Fragaria/Vitis*, based on the leaves of strawberries and vines; its real name is *Hepatodoron*, which means a *"donation, a gift, for the liver"*. It is an "archetypal remedy" of anthroposophic medicine and plays the role of harmonising the activity of the liver, put severely to the test by modern life. The doses of this humble, but precious remedy[66] will be prescribed by your doctor. I want to advise

---

[66] Dr. Aldo Bargero, the first Italian anthroposophic doctor, used to say ironically, but sincerely, that he should have had this remedy printed directly on his prescriptions. Recently we physicians and our patients have become aware of the importance of this remedy in a time when it is becoming impossible to find because of production problems. It had become the absolute centre of our little therapeutic nightmares and complaints from our patients.

you to have patience because this is absolutely not a laxative, but an ally of the liver which improves the performance of the digestive apparatus. The advice to chew the tablets is not given to make life more difficult, but to have an effect at a greater depth, stimulating the liver starting from the taste in the mouth. One last warning: this remedy contains lactose and is *contraindicated in people allergic to lactose*. Personally, I prescribe it with satisfaction to patients who suffer from a generic milk intolerance, because treating the liver means improving our relationship with the world that penetrates us through what we eat.

One precious remedy in line with this philosophy is *Cuprum 0.4% ointment*. Massaging this on the abdomen in a clockwise direction in the morning represents a message of movement; this ointment gives us the strength of copper, the remedy that combats cramps and stasis. If we want to make this treatment even more dynamic we can massage the insides of the legs with it in the evening, starting from the insides of the ankles and going up to the groin.

If we are lazy, in the evening we can simply massage the soles of the feet with copper, particularly the central part of the foot, which has a functional relationship with the abdomen.

If we suffer from venous insufficiency, as constipated people typically do, we can use *Cuprum 0.4%* on the abdomen in the morning and *Venadoron*[67] in the evening.

I recommend that the diet contains *flavourings*, which have the benefit of stimulating the activity of the internal organs (such as the salivary glands, stomach and duodenum), the production of bile and pancreatic juices and the activity of the intestinal bacterial flora.

Drink at least *six to eight glasses of water* each day; the water should not be cold and it is very useful to distribute this intake evenly throughout the day.

It is an excellent habit to drink a glass of *warm water in the morning*, when you wake up.

---

[67] Also called *Lotio pruni comp. cum Cupro*, a skin tonic that contains copper.

The old advice of *sitting on the lavatory in the morning* at a fixed time, preferably after breakfast, and of performing at least some physical activity, is justified. Common sense does, however, teach us not to transform this advice into an obsession which paralyses the metabolism and makes the bathroom inaccessible to the rest of the family.

The mysterious encopresis
Encopresis is defined as involuntary defecation in inappropriate places, at least once a month for three months or more in a child of four years old or more. It is a symptom that should be discussed with a doctor; it is usually the expression of some form of distress and to some extent the reflections in the chapter on bedwetting can be useful. These are always problems related to a weakness of the astral body in the metabolism which require education.

Haemorrhoids and anal fissures

Haemorrhoids
Haemorrhoids (piles) are dilatations of the submucosal veins of the anus and rectum (haemorrhoidal venous plexus) accompanied by an inflammatory reaction of the surrounding connective tissue. They may give no problems but are often manifested by loss of blood after the patient has passed a motion, a sense of heaviness, swelling, discomfort or itching, inflammation and pain in the anus, all typical of the acute inflammation.
Haemorrhoids may be *internal* if the dilatation[68] involves the veins above the anal sphincter or *external* if the dilatation concerns the haemorrhoidal plexus below the sphincter.
Chronic bleeding due to haemorrhoids can lead to severe anaemia. For this reason, I recommend that you tell your doctor

---

[68] In essence, haemorrhoids are varicose veins of the rectal venous system and, being without valves, become dilated with an increase in venous congestion in the region. The pressure within the abdomen is increased by *defecation, coughing, pregnancy* (a period during which haemorrhoids develop easily), *sneezing, vomiting, physical efforts* and by an increase in the pressure in the portal vein that carries blood to the liver; this increase in pressure is typical of cirrhosis of the liver (*portal hypertension*): it is for this reason that the old school of medicine rightly said that the presence of haemorrhoids means that the liver is tired and congested. It was said that there is *hepatic impairment*, a now outmoded term, such that a doctor expressing himself in this way risks appearing uninformed. If the liver is in difficulty, for example, when it receives an avalanche of chocolate via the portal vein, it unloads its congestion on the haemorrhoidal plexus, as gluttons of chocolate know well. Anybody who would like some illuminating reading on the subject of "scientific negation of reality" and on "how reality takes revenge on theories", should read the wonderful short story *L'invenzione del cavallo* by Achille Campanile, which describes the presentation of a supposedly new invention, the horse, to an audience of scientists. This invention creates amazement and envy among the scientists until a regiment of grenadiers on horseback passes by; at this point, the scientists, realising that the horse is not a new invention and that they have been teased, attack the poor inventor. I dedicate my affectionate thoughts to this neglected Italian master of the theatre of the absurd, certain that even in heaven, where he now lives, he will find grist for his humoristic mill.

if you have problems in this area, overcoming a reticence that has very old roots[69].

Dietary factors again

Haemorrhoids are a disorder of western society; in fact, they are rarely seen in those parts of the world where the diet is rich in fibre and unrefined foods. A diet poor in fibre and rich in processed foods strongly facilitates the development of haemorrhoids.

Paradoxically, those peoples that are not embarrassed to talk about haemorrhoids do not suffer from them; I am thinking about oriental peoples and their yoga, which deals with the hygiene and equilibrium of this area. In contrast, Americans and Europeans, as a result of the low content of fibre in their diet, tend to have to strain more during defecation, since their stools, being less bulky and more compact, are more difficult to expel. This straining increases pressure within the abdomen, preventing return of the blood. The higher intra-abdominal pressure increases pelvic congestion and can weaken the veins considerably, leading to the formation of haemorrhoids.

A diet rich in fibre is the most important strategy for preventing haemorrhoids. Fruit eaten with its skin, local vegetables that are in season, pulses and wholemeal cereals, all grown biodynamically (or biologically) promote intestinal peristalsis[70]; furthermore,

---

[69] We all know the hilarity and embarrassment that this subject creates. I discovered that one of my patients suffered from haemorrhoids only after having struggled to understand the cause of his severe anaemia. I remember accompanying him to the haematologist because we considered that he needed a transfusion. At the end I asked the right question and we were able to avoid the transfusion and a series of complex investigations aimed at discovering the cause of the bleeding, but he did require intravenous iron before he could be operated upon. I take the occasion to remind you that haemorrhoids are a surgical condition and when they are chronic and a certain degree of anatomo-pathological changes have occurred, they must be operated. Haemorrhoids are classified into *four stages of severity* and from the third stage are irreversible. At this point, we are grateful to surgery, which can lighten our life.

[70] *Intestinal peristalsis,* literally "contraction around", is a rhythmic and pro-

the fibre present in these foods absorb water and form a gelatinous mass that adds weight and volume to the faecal mass, making it softer and easier to expel; at the same time the fibre provide nutrients and support for a healthy bacterial flora. This is just one more reason in favour of the use of biodynamic wholemeal cereals in the diet.

In the chapter on hypertension, another "disease of civilisation", you will read that the other important factor for preventing and treating haemorrhoids is to *avoid a sedentary lifestyle*; healthy movement is fundamental for avoiding excessive congestion in the pelvis. Haemorrhoids are also occupational disorders, affecting people who remain seated for many hours, such as lorry drivers and office staff.

Some simple advice

We will give some advice on how to relieve discomfort and pain in the case of acute haemorrhoidal inflammation. A medical consultation is necessary for the correct diagnosis to be made, particularly if the symptoms are violent or the loss of blood is considerable or completely painless. It would be truly terrible to confuse haemorrhoids with cancer of the bowel.

A *warm hip bath* is a useful treatment for congested haemorrhoids. A hip bath is partial immersion of the pelvic region in water at a temperature between 38°C and 40°C.

Hamamelis distillata 10% ointment is useful for decongestion; this is applied locally at least a couple of times a day after cleaning the area. There are excellent anthroposophic suppositories for the treatment of haemorrhoids, but for these remedies you must consult your doctor.

There are, however, also reliable oral remedies that reduce irritation and pain.

---

gressive contraction of the circular smooth muscle of the digestive tract starting from the mouth along the whole of the gastrointestinal tract. It has the function of mixing the chyme with the digestive juices in the small intestines and propelling the intestinal contents towards the colon.

Aesculus cortex, ethanol. Decoctum D3 drops: the horse chestnut is the sovereign remedy for inflamed haemorrhoids; the dose is 10 drops every two hours until improvement, then followed by 10 drops three times a day before the three meals.

Aloe D6 drops or *granules* are useful to strengthen the effect of the *Aesculus*; the *Aesculus* can be alternated with *Aloe* (10 drops or 5 granules) every hour. Subsequently, when the symptoms have diminished, the two remedies can be alternated every two hours for a few days. Once the symptoms have resolved, maintenance therapy should be continued for several weeks with *Aesculus* before the three meals and *Aloe* after them. This is an effective treatment. *Aloe* is not available as an anthroposophic preparation, but can be found as a homeopathic product.

Achillea comp. drops. This is a very complete and useful compound remedy. Personally I use it for real treatment of the underlying problem; indeed, it contains *Achillea* and it was Rudolf Steiner himself who indicated that this plant, already known for other uses, is very important for the treatment of the liver. The dose is 10 drops every two or three hours for a few days to relieve the congestion and then 10 drops three times a day before the three meals.

Local hygiene and anal fissures

I advise against using soap to wash the anal area because it promotes swelling; personally I prescribe *Anonet pediatric*, a product for neonatal hygiene, although there are other valid products. It is very important not to use soap in the case of *anal fissures* or *anal rhagades*, which are long, linear lesions of the anal mucosa; these tend not to heal because of the trauma of defecation and the continual risk of infection. One typical symptom of anal fissures is pain during defecation which becomes very strong at the moment of passing the stools and lasts for as long as one or two hours. It is a condition that creates acute suffering, requires diagnosis and must be treated. A *fibre-rich diet* is indispensable and heals the condition in a large proportion of cases. In cases with strong *anal spasm* the use of *anal dilators* can be useful to promote healing of the wound; obviously this type of intervention should be prescribed by the doctor or specialist proctologist.

Calendula essence dilution for external use: 50 drops for a hip bath or in a bidet with tepid water. This is useful for disinfection and promoting formation of scar tissue. You should remain immersed for at least five minutes.

Calendula 20%/Echinacea 1% dilution for external use: this can be used in forms with burning and strong external inflammation. Use local compresses: soak a gauze in two fingers of lukewarm water to which 20 drops of the remedy have been added and apply the gauze to the affected area for at least ten minutes.

Calendula/Stibium cream: dry the region thoroughly and then apply the cream to the haemorrhoids and anal area.

Varicose veins and phlebitis

Varicose veins
Varicose veins are dilated, tortuous veins, mainly of the legs.
As described for haemorrhoids, they are caused by an increase in venous pressure, which occurs, for example, in pregnancy or in cases of work requiring standing upright on one's feet for many hours. This increase in pressure causes dilatation and bulging of the walls of the veins and damage to the valves of the veins, with a consequent downwards flow of the blood.
In the legs, the blood which would tend to flow downwards under the effect of gravity tends, instead, to be pushed upwards by the pumping activity of the muscles which rhythmically compress the deep veins, pushing the blood towards the heart; furthermore, the veins contain a system of internal valves that make the blood flow in only one direction, closing when the blood tends to flow back downwards. If the blood cannot move towards the heart and tends to pool within the veins as the result of failure of the valves, the increased pressure begins to stretch the walls of the vessels, causing varicose veins.
There is a considerable hereditary tendency to this disorder, which must be managed with an adequate lifestyle.
Risk factors are constipation (haemorrhoids and varicose veins are often associated), insufficient physical activity, work requiring long periods of standing, smoking, obesity, and a diet poor in roughage, fruit and vegetables (which contain factors that protect the circulation). The dietary recommendations given for haemorrhoids are also valid for varicose veins. Walking a certain distance each day promotes emptying of the veins and reduces venous pressure. One important remedy of varicose veins is horse chestnut, especially when the varicose veins are associated with haemorrhoids. This is, in any case, a problem that requires a disease-modifying treatment from the doctor, who must also be consulted in order to have a clear diagnosis. Here I limit myself to giving some brief advice.

Aesculus hippocastanum D6 granules or *D3 drops,* 3 granules or 10 drops before the three meals, for at least three months. This remedy can be considered both as a venous tonic with anti-inflammatory and anti-oedema activity as well as a general tonic which supports hepatic activity.
Aesculus gemme 1D macerated glycerol: derived from the buds of horse chestnut. This is a remedy that can be taken for a long time without risks; take 50 drops in the morning in a glass of water, for long periods. One strongly indicated background remedy, in cases in which varicose veins are associated with haemorrhoids, is *Borago comp. globules,* 10 globules before the three meals, as a long-term treatment; this is a remedy which is prescribed to stimulate the formative forces and blood flow.
Venadoron (Lotio pruni comp. cum Cupro): this is an excellent remedy to apply in the evening with a light massage to the inner parts of the legs starting from the ankles up to the groin; it is very pleasant in the summer when the legs are tired.

Post-traumatic phlebitis
In post-traumatic phlebitis, a localised venous inflammation occurring as a result of trauma or strong contusion of a vein, Hamamelis (witch-hazel) is particularly indicated and we can consider it the "arnica for the veins".
Apply *Hamamelis distillate ointment 10%* locally and cover with a light dressing. This ointment is very useful for localised venous inflammation.
In post-traumatic inflammation, a combination of *Hamamelis, ethanol. Decoctum (cortex) D3 drops* can be used: take 10 drops, in a little water, every two or three hours for the first days following the trauma, continuing for at least ten days, taking 10 drops before the three meals.

A gift from the animal world: leeches
For over twenty years I have used leeches for the specific treatment of varicose veins, to the satisfaction of my patients. This is an excellent treatment because the leeches, in order to be able to

use blood that they suck from a person, inject substances that work as anticoagulants and carry out a useful role of decongesting the surrounding venous site; furthermore, when sucking blood, the leech exerts a very healthy traction on the veins. Leeches have come back into favour also in conventional medicine, in which they are used mainly in refined reconstructive surgery, because they effectively counteract post-operative swelling and oedema. On July 12, 2004, the American Food and Drug Administration authorised the marketing of leeches for medical use in the United States of America, where they are used in skin grafting and in reconstructive surgery in hospitals.

I have mentioned this subject of leeches because I believe that there is no reason why everything that has a long history and is the fruit of great experience should be hastily abandoned as outdated. Of course the leeches must be applied directly by an expert doctor after clinical and laboratory examinations have been carried out; I am strongly against a "do-it-yourself" approach, since a leech applied to the wrong site or on weakened tissue can cause an ulcer which is then difficult to heal. Finally, the leeches should be bought in pharmacies that guarantee that they are purchased from a suitable breeding centre. Since these are animals that feed on blood, care is needed. Our time gives us some concerns but also some certainties that we must not renounce

Leeches and post-partum phlebitis

One last consideration: I know of no other treatment that is as cost-effective and fast as the application of two or three leeches in the case of *acute phlebitis*. I have had wonderful experiences of this treatment in the case of *post-partum venous inflammation*: the problem is resolved quickly and the patient can continue to breastfeed without problems.

A change of air

I want to use this popular, old expression, better suited to us Europeans and with a broader meaning than Americanisms such as *jet-lag*, to indicate that state of psycho-physical adaptation required after a journey; a state that may last from a few hours to several days, depending on the extent of the journey and individual predisposition. A type of medical care the vocation of which is "accompanying the human being as he is manifested" spurns no signs and finds it noble to deal with even the most humble of symptoms.

Onopordon/Primula comp. drops. One excellent help comes from a remedy for the heart (conceived by Steiner as "*Cardiodoron*", or a gift, a friend for the heart[71]). During and, above all, after a journey, the body needs to adapt to the change, which occurs extremely rapidly thanks to modern means of transport, without the heart having the possibility of perceiving the magnitude of the shift on the Earth's surface. This remedy helps the heart gain confidence with the new situation. The dose is 10 drops before the three meals, in a little water, starting two or three days before departure and continuing for at least one week after returning. When the journey is followed by a certain period at the destination, you can stop taking the drops and then start taking them again before returning.

This remedy supports the heart, balances the heart-lung rhythm[72]

---

[71] These specific remedies which end with the suffix "doron", such as *Pneumodoron*, *Kephalodoron* or *Renodoron*, are called "archetypal remedies" because they are designed as a gift, a donation, for the organ, or for a function or to tackle an illness. In some countries, for legal reasons, these remedies cannot always be referred to by these invented names and are, therefore, described by the names of their main constituents, such as *Aconitum/Bryonia* for *Pneumodoron 1*, a remedy for bronchitis.

[72] The relationship between the basic rhythm of the lungs, ideally 18 breaths per minute, and the heart, at 72 beats per minute, is a balanced ratio of one to four, which is considered an important sign of health in an anthroposophic clinical examination.

and helps the senses to become accustomed to the new environment.

Travel and intestinal activity
We owe Rudolf Steiner for the information that hunger, that is, the need for solid food, is regulated by the lungs. This knowledge clarifies why we have such important dietary changes in the case of severe disorders of the lungs, such as loss of appetite in the case of tuberculosis, and also explains the high risk of lung disorders in pathologically thin individuals, who have an exasperated desire to "become ethereal", that is, to refuse to take part of the earth with the help of solid food. Some bitter foods, such as Icelandic lichen (see the chapter on cough), bring us back into our body through the lungs. We can recognize this from the fact that the appetite returns, the "desire to connect with the earth" comes back. The link between the lungs and the earth is even evident in the case of chronic lung disorders, when it is precisely the "change of air" that is exploited: for example, the seaside to surround a patient by iodine, salt and silica. In contrast, patients with pulmonary tuberculosis are taken to breathe the air of the high mountains, where the granite and powerful forces of the light can act as formative forces in the lungs. This explains why some lung disorders cannot be treated in certain parts of the Earth and only a change of location can provide the definitive cure for the illness. This is to say that in an age like ours, when new viral diseases, such as atypical pneumonias[73], are occurring and creating panic, it would be very useful to listen to anthroposophic knowledge and invest in research aimed at creating a future geographical medicine. However, let us go back to simple tourist trips. A change of air is notorious for playing a role in slowing intestinal activity which, in the light of modern understanding of the immunological system, means a weakening in the

---

[73] SARS (an acronym for severe acute respiratory syndrome), or atypical pneumonia, is a disease related to new interactions between previously harmless viruses that have now, as a result of a mutation, become very dangerous.

A change of air

body's defence mechanisms. The ease with which we fall ill so often during travel is also due to the temporary inactivity of the most important of our defence organs, that is, the intestine. All the currents of medicine that consider functional and energy interactions between organs know of the profound relationship between the lungs, the organ through which the "new air" resulting from travel penetrates the body, and the colon, the organ that slows its own activity to avoid overloading the lungs. It was precisely this relationship between the intestines and the lungs that led ancient Hippocratic medicine to use enemas to treat disorders of the airways, as we have already said when discussing the sore throat. Our grandmothers were right when they said you need to "clean" the intestines after a journey!

The best treatment for the metabolism is still the old purge that our mothers and grandmothers gave us at every arrival at our holiday destination and at every return home. The traditional *castor oil*, taken in the evening before going to bed, is certainly still a valid solution. For individuals with delicate bowels, or for children more than four to six years old, a generous dose of *Fragaria/Vitis tablets*, an archetypal remedy for the liver, may be sufficient on its own. The recommended treatment is to chew 3 tablets from three to six times a day. Half doses are used for children (1 tablet three to six times a day).

I have used this remedy successfully even in people at risk of diarrhoea, giving some dietary advice together with the *Fragaria/Vitis*. Indeed, our holidays often become a nightmare because the "all inclusive" formula leads us to lose our common sense, which is always the best prevention.

Simply as an example I would like to remind you that in Abruzzo alone, just a single region of the wonderful country of Italy, there are over 50 organic or biodynamic tourist farms where, spending less than you would in a holiday village, you can eat organic food while staying in a healthy, instructive and peaceful environment. Perhaps it would be worth us all reflecting on those holidays from which we return home more tired, stressed and unhappy than before we left.

Enuresis: the wet bed

Nocturnal enuresis is the involuntary loss of urine during the night in a child of five years old or upwards, in the absence of particular illnesses.
Classical enuresis is characterized by only nocturnal symptoms and accounts for 85% of cases. The condition is called primary if the child has never been dry at night for more than six months and secondary if the child starts wetting his bed again after having been dry at night for at least six months.
From 15-20% of children aged 5 years old, 7% of those 7 years old, 5% of 10-year olds, 2-3% of children between 12 and 14 years old, and 1-2% of the population of individuals 15 years old and over wet their bed on average twice a week. About 15% of children with enuresis stop bed-wetting spontaneously, without treatment, within one year.
These data help me to give a little comfort to parents of bed-wetters; they must have trust, because the condition almost always resolves spontaneously. There is often some family history; the father of a bed-wetter very probably had the same problem and remembering this often forgotten fact can help to overcome the lack of faith. Enuresis is a disorder that severely tasks the patience of the parents, but is also frustrating for the affected child. I should say immediately that isolated episodes of bed-wetting, for example once or twice a month, are of minimal clinical relevance because they probably simply reflect an anxious nature or an emotional response to stressful events. I recommend parents a certain *"art" of nappy use* because attempts to resolve the problem with force, with rages or with violent punishments will do no other than worsen the frustration and the disorder, strongly risking making it become chronic. I am convinced that adults suffering from enuresis hide a severe family problem going back to infancy, which requires a real "spiritual journey" to be overcome. I remember one of the most engaging "adventures" of my medical experience was just such a journey I undertook together with an

Enuresis: the wet bed

adult who had disconsolately confessed his problem to me.

Often an early, forced gain of control of the bladder in a child and early abandonment of nappies create the basis for future bed-wetting, which may occur after years, for example when starting infant school or junior school[74]. Modern nappies that are so absorbent (and so polluting to the environment!) do not cause that natural discomfort that facilitates the achievement of bladder control. Sometimes, before ceasing to use nappies suddenly, it can be useful to change to a less comfortable nappy.

The other aspect of this parental "art" consists in the right *appeal to the forces of will*. Attempts must be made to stimulate the child to use his will to control his bladder, giving him moral encouragement, that is giving praise and attention to his efforts, dedicating a little, but precious time to rewarding a night passed without bed-wetting. Children ask for toys and sweets as rewards, only because they do not know that they could be more gratified by adults worthy of their love. Nothing of a consumerist mirage can replace the profound interest of an adult in a child! I have had the experience of seeing children living in institutes, inundated with toys of every sort, who had enormous and lifelong benefits from being put into a foster family which spent even just a few minutes teaching them how to look after their own body or to use cutlery at the table; a video game has no benefit for either the sight or the nervous system. Dear readers, allow me to repeat, once again, that a real educator is great and accomplished when he demonstrates the respect he has for the person he is educating.

Anthroposophic medicine has excellent remedies for helping a child with enuresis, so put your trust in your doctor who should not, however, absolve you from working on *respect as a force that feeds the self-will* of your children and of other children that you have the fortune to meet.

---

[74] With regards to enuresis, Rudolf Steiner spoke of weakness of the astral body and stated that in certain cases a child could be cured by moral actions, simply reinforcing his attention to his own bodily functions.

Some simple advice for strengthening the astral body
Here are some useful tips: do not give your child anything to drink after a certain hour in the evening, try to make him move enough to sweat during the day, avoid stimuli to the abdomen such as constipation or heavy blankets, teach him to empty his bladder completely and, perhaps, give him a small alarm clock when he is a little bit older, so that he can remain dry on particular occasions such as staying overnight at a friend's house.

Reducing the number of wet nights and decreasing the effect of bed-wetting on a child's lifestyle can contribute to creating a favourable background for the much desired nocturnal continence. If we parents don't believe in ourselves, how can a child believe in us? Do not allow yourself to be beaten by cynicism – a mortal disease. Don't be ashamed to be joyful for one dry night. Laugh with joy for a dry bed!

Cystitis and urethritis

Cystitis

The urinary tract is sterile and very resistant to invasion by bacteria but, as a fascinating paradox of the human state, infection of the urinary tract is one of the most common bacterial infections in all age groups. Cystitis[75] is an inflammation of the bladder and is almost always caused by bacteria; nevertheless, urine is a naturally sterile solution that counteracts the development of bacteria thanks to its physiologically high concentrations of urea and salts. It is known that urine is an excellent disinfectant, used from time immemorial in popular medicine to treat sores, skin lesions and burns.

What often makes urine a suitable medium for the development of pathogenic flora is the ecological imbalance created by the *contemporary lifestyle,* by continuous exposure to artificially cooled and heated environments, by *industrialised nutrition* containing substances that irritate and thin the mucosa of the bladder, but above all, by *repeated courses of antibiotics.* A rational treatment must aim to restore the biological balance between our body and the bacterial flora that it houses.

Despite its striking achievements, modern biomolecular medicine, based on the mistaken conception that the laws that govern mineral matter can mechanically be applied to living beings, leads us to the unpleasant consequence of physically experiencing, with stinging pain in the urinary tract, the difference between the laws of the physical world and the laws of the etheric world of life. In fact, according to a purely physical logic, *Escherichia coli,* responsible for 80% of urinary tract infections, should disappear when exposed to antibiotics, but in the world of real life, in the etheric, the principle of metamorphosis applies so that, precisely as the result of repeated antibiotic treatment, this formidable and

---

[75] Cystitis, from the Greek *kyst(is)* ("bladder"), and *itis* ("inflammation"), or "inflammation of the bladder".

wondrous bacillus is transformed from a normal, friendly inhabitant of the intestine (as its very name tells us: *coli* means "colon dweller"), which produces almost all the group B vitamins[76] that our body needs, into an enemy invader and destroyer of the urinary mucosa.

In recent years, cystitis has responded ever less well to antibiotics, even though, as we have had already said, 80% of cases are caused by *Escherichia coli*. This is because this bacterium has learnt to manufacture resistance factors to antibiotics and also to transmit this capacity for resistance to other bacteria, through particles of DNA called plasmids[77]. Clinical experience has taught us that it is increasingly difficult to treat recurrent episodes of cystitis after the first miraculous successes achieved with antibiotics. Indeed, experts in infectious diseases have expressed concern about this problem. In my clinical practice I often see people who have come to me after years of repeated episodes of cystitis, sometimes with one attack following another by only one or two months. These people have a really poor quality of life. Furthermore, there are women who have cystitis after every sexual intercourse with their own and only partner. Although we know that the incidence of bacteriuria (bacteria in the urine) is much lower among nuns, a monastic life certainly cannot be the solution to the problem for everyone.

---

[76] This is the reason why doctors combine a group B multivitamin with a prescription for antibiotics; in fact, for a certain period the intestinal bacterial flora will not be able to carry out its task of producing these vitamins.

[77] A *plasmid*, or *plasmidium*, is a particle present in the cytoplasm of many bacteria which contains genetic material that is not part of chromosomes. During bacterial conjugation, plasmids are passed from one bacterium to another and the transfer of the genes in these plasmids is involved in *resistance to antibiotics* or the production of bacteriocins or toxins. Many natural or partially synthesised plasmids are used in *genetic engineering* as cloning vectors, that is, they are part of *recombinant DNA techniques* in which a specific sequence of DNA is inserted into an appropriate vector, with the aim of propagating numerous copies through the reproduction of the cells into which the vector has been introduced. *Col plasmids* are plasmids containing genes that command the production of bacteriocins, known as colicins, against *Escherichia coli* and other species of bacteria. Some *Col plasmids* may also carry resistance genes.

As far as concerns children, we must remember that faced with a high fever of sudden onset, without either pain or a cough, we must always consider an infection of the kidneys or cystitis, particularly in babies and young children, in whom cystitis is painless. Thus, the first thing to do in the case of a young child with a fever without an apparent cause is to examine the urine in order to help clarify the diagnosis.

However, the urine must also always be examined in adults, in the presence of symptoms such as a continuous desire to pass urine and a burning sensation or pain in the lower abdomen, which may spread to the groin and the anus. The urine must be collected in the morning after having carefully cleaned and abundantly rinsed the external genitals and having discarded the first stream of urine. The urine should be collected into a sterile container, which can be bought from a chemist's shop. The request for a *urine culture*, which serves to identify the microbes involved, must include an *antibiogram* to determine the most effective antibiotic for that particular microbe. In this way the doctor can select the most appropriate treatment. Often a patient does not go to the doctor early enough, but waits until the symptoms are very severe, which forces the physician to prescribe a treatment immediately, which will not be specific for that patient's particular infection.

Initial acute cystitis
It is interesting to know that the two great remedies for febrile colds, *Aconitum* and *Belladonna*, are very effective in initial acute cystitis, demonstrating that cystitis is strongly related to the warmth body, as I shall explain later on.
Aconitum D6 drops or *granules*: these are useful for acute, sudden-onset cystitis, characterized by violent symptoms, widespread pain and difficulty in urinating; the patient is anxious, frightened, very restless and pale, has cold shivers, dry skin and is very thirsty. This sort of cystitis is caused by having caught cold, especially from having been exposed to cold wind, when a person is warm, but may also result from a fright.

Part II. Illnesses and remedies

Belladonna D6 drops or *granules*: this is another remedy that is useful in an immediately acute, strong, sudden and violent cystitis, accompanied in this case by marked sweating and congestion of the face; the patient is aggressive and not very thirsty. Tenesmus[78] of the bladder and fluid retention develop rapidly.

One or other of the two remedies named above can be used: the doses are 10 drops or 3 granules every two hours for *Aconitum*, the therapeutic effects of which are completed with strong sweating, and every hour for *Belladonna*, the action of which is useful for a longer period. This is a treatment for the initial stage of the disorder, and can even resolve the problem if used at the onset of the very first signs.

Aconitum comp. globules: these globules contain the three great remedies for febrile colds: *Aconitum D30*, *Belladonna D30*, *Rhus toxicodendron D30*. It is a remedy designed for neuralgias and neuritis, but which can be of help in diagnostically uncertain cases and when there is doubt as to whether to use *Aconitum* or *Belladonna*, while waiting for the doctor's assessment. The dose is 10 globules every one or two hours.

Berberis/Apis comp. globules: these contain *Belladonna* and *Apis*, the two major remedies for inflammation, besides *Berberis* for the throat and *Terebinthina* for urinary tract irritation, two remedies that are in any case specific for the urinary tract. The composite remedy stimulates the warmth body and harmonises the altered interaction between the astral and ether bodies, typical of inflammation of the bladder, but also of the mouth (stomatitis) and frontal sinuses (sinusitis, which, like cystitis, is an illness due to cold); once again we can see that the warmth body is at the centre of his disorder. This remedy can be used in cases of initial cystitis that start slowly and gradually (a moderate cystitis that is not violent, as described for *Belladonna* and *Aconitum*) with burning and discomfort only during urination. The dose is 10 globules

---

[78] "Tenesmus" of the bladder, from the Greek *teinein* ("to stretch, strain"), is the spasmodic contraction of the bladder sphincter associated with a constant desire to urinate, although only small amounts of urine may be passed or none at all.

every two hours; as usual, the remedy should not be withdrawn immediately, but should be tapered down gradually, first to every three hours and then to every four hours for a few days.

Cantharis comp. globules: this is a remedy for a cystitis that worsens over a few hours, with intense pain during but also after having urinated. The medical prescription in the case of cystitis that becomes very painful and in which blood appears in the urine (haematuria) is the same remedy injected subcutaneously; this is a very effective therapy if given in that area of the belly. It should be used while waiting for the results of examinations and the definitive decision of the doctor.

In less severe cases, *Berberis/Apis globules* can be used: 10 globules every one or two hours.

One criterion for choosing is the following: *Cantharis* is more appropriate for persistent burning and pain, up to the point of violent symptoms such as tenesmus, while *Berberis* is more suitable for irritation and discomfort while urinating. In the forms with mixed symptoms, the two remedies can be alternated: 10 globules of one of the two remedies every one or two hours.

I shall describe three more useful remedies to choose from, depending on the different symptoms related to urination; use 10 drops every two or three hours, possibly combining two of the remedies described:

Equisetum arvense D6 drops: to be used in the case of abundant urine with pain particularly at the end of urination;

Staphysagria D6 drops: to be used in cases of burning pain, felt in particular in the interval between passing urine and which improves clearly or even stops during urination itself;

Cantharis D4 drops: to be used for violent pain which worsens immediately before, during and after voiding a generally small volume of urine. Blood, even large amounts, may be present in the urine after several hours.

As far as concerns healthy living measures to apply during an episode of cystitis, the recommendations are to drink a lot, reduce the amount of food intake and have a light diet, as for all acute illnesses.

For advice on footbaths and hip baths, see the chapter on colds. I always recommend a good *tea* based on equal doses of *bearberries, horsetail, couch grass* and *yarrow*. Pour a heaped teaspoon of the mixture into a cup of boiling water, cover the cup and leave to steep for ten minutes and then filter. It can be useful to prepare a litre of the tea using two tablespoons of the mixture and keep it in a large flask, drinking it throughout the day.

Recurrent cystitis
This form of cystitis is a real scourge. Remedies are not sufficient to cure it, and work must be done on the person's lifestyle. It is essential to *treat the warmth body*. Avoid clothes made from artificial fibres, use socks, trousers and underwear of pure wool. Be careful not to wear clothes that are too short and not to lose warmth from the hands and in particular from the feet. The zones at risk for cystitis are the soles of the feet, the ankles, the area of the "waist" and the lower abdomen. Woollen pants can be very effective in children, even in the case of a so-called "weak bladder", that is, when there is a tendency to cystitis. Walking barefoot on cold floors in the house is risky behaviour in individuals predisposed to cystitis. I think we all know that the cause of cystitis in the late summer is walking barefoot in the night on the beaches and/or in the morning on campsite grass. Experience teaches us that it is very difficult to recover from a chronic cystitis while scuttling around on a moped with the waist exposed to wind or when wearing slippers in damp places; this shows us just how important it is to look after our own warmth.

One good treatment for recurrent cystitis is a *hot footbath* in the evening in order to provide warmth. The treatment can be made more specific for the bladder by pouring a large cup of *equisetum tea* into the footbath. In anthroposophic medicine, equisetum is a plant for treating the kidneys; a cup of the tea can also be drunk to carry the protective effect of the silica in the equisetum into the metabolic sphere (see also *hip baths*).

Preparation: in the morning pour a tablespoon of *equisetum* (popularly called *horsetail*) into half a litre of water, leave to macerate for twelve hours, bring to boil and then filter. Drink a glass and use the rest for the footbath. Of course the tea can also be prepared as a normal infusion in boiling water, particularly if we have forgotten to prepare it in the morning, although with the foresight of leaving the horsetail in the infusion for half an hour, then filtering it and, perhaps, warming it again. The long period of infusion serves to make a breach in the silica covering that forms the skeleton and support of this time-honoured, reliable plant.

Drink a lot! This is important to keep the urinary tract in balance at all times, but it is *absolutely essential to avoid cold drinks*. You will realise just how "un-human" it is to drink and eat cold things: for example, a cold alcoholic drink facilitates cystitis just as much as cold milk promotes the development of diarrhoea.

Kalium/Teucrium comp. dilution: this is a background remedy for a tendency to recurrent cystitis, to strengthen the mucosa and make it less fragile and irritable, and to help the local equilibrium of the warmth body which suffers from cooling, but also from sudden increases of heat caused, for example, by foods that "irritate, through warming" such as chocolate and alcoholic drinks, "the fire water" of native Americans. A suggested dose is 10 to 15 drops before the three meals; the treatment should be continued for a long period.

It is important to strengthen the peripheral boundary that the etheric substance tends not to have.

Sometimes *external treatments* are therapeutically effective precisely because of this fundamental law. Until recently we successfully used baths of *Formica rufa for external use*, which unfortunately is no longer available: it is not only the great panda that is disappearing, but also our best remedies! I regret this, but it becomes an occasion not to be repetitive in our treatments.

I advise at least *warm hip baths* (immerging the body up to the navel) pouring two spoonfuls of *Equisetum arvense dilution for external use* into the bath and stirring the water well. This preparation is also excellent for footbaths, in which case only one spoonful should be used.

After the hip bath, the lower abdomen can be massaged with *Formica 1% ointment*.
This treatment can be carried out two or three times a week for at least three months.

Interstitial cystitis
Interstitial cystitis deserves a separate discussion. This new term, which has spread through the world, has finally given formal recognition to what wise doctors have always known, that the underlying cause of cystitis is never the microbes but is inherent to what natural medicine calls the "terrain": in a certain sense we can consider that the *warmth* which we are always speaking of in anthroposophic medicine represents the *humus*, the living component of the earth; in this way we can study the physiology of the bladder from a completely new angle and finally understand the formidable work that this organ plays in the human body. I shall repeat myself once again, saying that there is no such thing as a local disease! It is always the human being as a whole who becomes ill. Of course it is clear that the apparently simple recurrent cystitis due to *Escherichia coli* is actually the expression of a colibacillosis, in other words an important problem of the intestinal flora that must be treated with a good diet and lifestyle and, possibly, complex remedies to restore intestinal symbiosis.

I report here some notes on the definition from the Interstitial Cystitis Association (ICA)[79]:
– "*Interstitial cystitis is a chronic inflammatory condition of the bladder the cause of which is still unknown. 'Common' cystitis, also known as a urinary tract infection, is normally treated with antibiotics with a positive outcome. Unlike common cystitis, interstitial cystitis is not considered to be caused by bacteria and does not respond to conventional treatment with antibiotics. It is important to note that interstitial cystitis is not a psychosomatic disorder and is not caused by stress. Interstitial cystitis can affect people of any*

[79] See the website: *www.ichelp.org*.

age, race or gender. However, women are affected much more frequently. Recent epidemiological data seem to indicate that there are over 700,000 cases in the USA. Some or all of the following symptoms may be present in cases of interstitial cystitis:
FREQUENCY: frequent urination (up to 60 times a day in severe cases) during the day and/or night. This is sometimes the only symptom of the condition in very mild cases or in the initial stages.
URGENCY: the impellent need to urinate, which can be accompanied by pain, a sense of pressure or spasms.
PAIN: can be localised to the area of the lower abdomen, urethra or vagina. Furthermore, the pain is frequently associated with sexual intercourse. Men affected by interstitial cystitis may have pain in the testicles, scrotum and/or perineum and find ejaculation painful.
OTHER DISORDERS: besides the more widespread symptoms of interstitial cystitis listed above, some patients report also having muscle and joint pains, migraines, allergic reactions and gastrointestinal problems. It also seems that interstitial cystitis is associated, in a not completely understood manner, with some painful syndromes such as vulvar vestibulitis, fibromyalgia and irritable bowel syndrome. However, many patients with interstitial cystitis only have bladder symptoms".
– "Many people with interstitial cystitis consider that food plays an important role in helping them to control the condition and avoid acute exacerbations. Others do not think that what they eat or drink has any effect on their state. If you have not already tried changing your own diet, we advise you to experiment with different foods and drinks to see whether this approach works".
– "Avoid beer, wine, spirits, coffee, seasoned cheeses, yeast, dried or cured meats, artificial sweeteners and fizzy drinks. Use decaffeinated coffee and tea with reduced acidity. Drink still mineral water rather than tap water".
– "Follow a diet with low acidity, eliminating foods such as tomatoes, vinegar, mayonnaise, ketchup, mustard, citrus fruits, fruit juices or products that contain these ingredients".
– "Avoid spicy foods and chocolate (which contains caffeine)".

*– "Add unprocessed fibre to your diet to promote regular bowel movements".
– "Do not smoke".
– "Eat several small meals instead of a single large one".
– "Some studies have indicated that a dietary supplement containing calcium glycerophosphate, when used with food and drinks with a high acid content by people who suffer from interstitial cystitis, helps to reduce bladder pain and the sensation of an impellent need to urinate".*

Personally, having studied this problem, which has long been ignored by conventional medicine that is always searching for the microbe involved, I have realised that anthroposophic medicine offers great opportunities. This is because some of the suggestions that have been "discovered" by this voluntary organisation are extended in our clinical practice, but above all, can be seen in context and understood. I am convinced that I have treated this condition when I still could not give it a precise name. I encourage you to consult your anthroposophic doctor for such an important problem.

Urethritis
Urethritis is an acute or chronic inflammatory process of the urethra, the last part of the urinary tract, and is almost always associated with cystitis (urethrocystitis). The specific forms, such as gonococcal, tubercular or syphilitic urethritis are beyond the scope of these reflections.
Here I shall discuss the so-called non-specific urethritis, a common urinary tract infection caused by the bacterial flora resident in the urethra which can become unbalanced for various reasons such as minute trauma, pregnancy, abortion, instrumental investigations and diabetes. *Escherichia coli* is very frequently involved, as in the more common cases of cystitis. The symptoms include a purulent discharge, difficulty in urinating and a tendency to pass little urine, but often. The margins of the urinary outlet are swollen and reddened.

Cystitis and urethritis

In males, urethritis is often associated with epididymitis (an inflammation of the epididymis, a duct of the testicles) by extension of the infection to the posterior urethra. In women, the infection almost always involves the cervix as well as the urethra and, sometimes, also the vaginal fornix.

If the symptoms are not too severe, you can start to treat the infection with the remedies used for cystitis, although always performing at least a bacterial examination of the urine and urinary sediment, in order that your doctor can have all the information necessary. It is essential that you undergo this investigation before you start taking an antibiotic.

The treatment and defence of our warmth are also important for urethritis: warm footbaths, keeping the lower abdomen covered and wearing thick socks are always very useful behaviours both in the acute stage and to avoid possible recurrences.

Menstrual pain (dysmenorrhoea)

We can say that the different forms of dysmenorrhoea are not an inevitable curse for women, but can be tackled and, in many cases, resolved brilliantly.

Even at the age of full fertility, menstruation is frequently preceded or accompanied by pelvic pain (pain in the lower abdomen), lumbo-sacral (back) pain, migraine and vomiting, especially at the start of the cycle but also often in the following period.

This is a situation in which the astral body intervenes too intensely in the physical body, triggering a state of consciousness in an erroneous place, in other words, pain. A remedy working specifically on the condition is useful and necessary, although in certain very acute cases common "over-the-counter" analgesics can be effective. For instance, I have prescribed such analgesics for school trips or when adolescents go abroad, leaving the specific treatment for when they return. I certainly do, therefore, advise that you consult your own anthroposophic doctor, who will prescribe a treatment aimed particularly at regulating the cycle and flow.

For example, an archetypal remedy for regulating the menstrual cycle is *Capsella/Majorana comp.*, a mixture of plants that stimulate the flow and others that block it, thus promoting the creation of a sort of "little pelvic woman" in the etheric within the female body; this "little pelvic woman" provides functional support as a faithful friend would do. More than a drug, we can consider it as a gift to female function.

A good symptomatic remedy is *Belladonna/Chamomilla globules*. I advise taking 10 globules before the three meals for some days before menstruation in order to create a favourable condition for the bleeding itself.

If you suffer from *premenstrual syndrome* (agitation, irritability, bloating, breast pain), take the globules from the time of ovulation up to the menstrual period, combining them with the capsules of *Primula Oenothera biennis (evening primrose)*, one in the morning and one in the evening for two or three months. The oil extracted from the seeds of this plant, which is common in meadows, contains gamma-linolenic acid (an essential fatty acid), a precursor of the prostaglandins involved in inflammatory processes.

The common analgesics act precisely as anti-prostaglandins. The difference lies in the fact that with anthroposophic treatment we do not try to eliminate the prostaglandins, but to promote the formation of anti-inflammatory prostaglandins and suppress the inflammatory ones: "we teach" the body the right actions.

Of course a good diet obtains a very profound effect, as can be seen from the low incidence of premenstrual syndrome among populations that eat healthy foods rich in essential fatty acids, such as the seeds and oils of linseed, sunflower and maize, sesame and biological sesame butter (tahini), herbs, soy, almonds, walnuts, and biodynamic olive oil.

Finally, a *tea of liquorice root* (two cups a day in the two weeks following ovulation) is an excellent aid to restoring the balance between oestrogens and progesterone, altered slightly in favour of the former in cases of premenstrual syndrome, and often also in dysmenorrhoea.

Returning to *Belladonna/Chamomilla*, once the first day of the menstrual period has been reached, at the very first sign of bleeding, take 5 granules every half hour, progressively reducing the frequency of administration only once the cycle is fully underway, in any case when the critical moment has passed.

Anthroposophic medicine teaches that many gynaecological problems, including dysmenorrhoea, are the long-term consequence of chronically cold feet, of which the patient has often lost awareness.

A good preventive measure, besides wearing *woollen socks during the cold season* and *not wearing synthetic fabrics*, is to use *alternating hot and cold footbaths*: one minute in hot water and 15 seconds in a bowl of cold water, to which a tablespoon of *Arnica essence for external use* has been added. Repeat the procedure a dozen times, carrying out the footbath at least three evenings a week.

Urania's copper insoles[80] are certainly a good help to warm the feet; it is recommended that they are used constantly for at least six months, not forgetting to transfer them from one pair of shoes to another.

---

[80] These are leather soles that are impregnated with copper, typical of the anthroposophic medical tradition. Copper is a classical anthroposophic remedy for spasms and a circulation weakened by the cold (see the chapter on muscle cramps).

Impetigo

Impetigo is a very contagious, superficial infection of the skin caused by bacteria. These bacteria are normally present on the skin but proliferate and cause the infection if the barrier function of the skin is impaired. It is precisely for this reason that impetigo is more common in the summer, when the skin is not covered and, therefore, more vulnerable.

The infection must be recognized and treated, both because it is very contagious – it can be caught just by touching the lesions or the hands of affected people – and to prevent any complications that could result from its spreading.

It usually starts at a point where the skin has been damaged, for example by an insect bite or a scratch: this is where vesicles or blisters form, surrounded by a red halo. The vesicles contain a clear liquid that becomes cloudy and burst easily, discharging a yellowy liquid that leads to the formation of a yellowish scab. The infection spreads quickly via the fingers and towels, so new lesions can develop at some distance from the original ones. Impetigo frequently affects children and is often transmitted to their mothers. The diagnosis is simple, the disorder is recognized easily and does not require particular investigations. The treatment must, however, be started immediately, be correct and be protracted in order to prevent the spread of the infection in the patient but also in his family and among his peers. If the infection occurs while the person is on holiday – as it often does – it is worth using traditional therapy based on thorough disinfection and local treatment with an antibiotic; finally, the lesions should be dressed carefully to prevent self-contagion and contagion of others. A general antibiotic only needs to be used in particularly extensive cases or in children with impaired defences.

If an illness has preceded the impetigo, this illness must also be treated. In fact it is common that impetigo develops on an existing lesion, for example, a scratch in someone with atopic eczema, or on repeated insect bites (see the chapter on bites and stings).

One piece of advice that I do think I can give is to clean the skin thoroughly with *Calendula essence* before medicating the lesions. It is worth having this natural detergent available always: it is very useful to apply a dilution of the essence, 10 to 15 drops in a quarter cup of water, to any type of skin lesion to help the barrier function of the skin. A compress moistened with diluted *Calendula* several times during the day can be tried as an initial treatment of localised impetigo, taking care to prevent self-contagion of the infection by carefully used dressings. Given the very contagious nature of this infection, it is also worth using different towels. The most frequently affected areas are the face, neck, hands and limbs. Children's nails should be cut regularly, particularly in the summer, and the children must be prevented from picking at the scabs. The treatment requires patience and perseverance.

Calendula ointment 10% is less effective in the initial stage but can be used when the lesions start to recede. A good remedy to administer after the compress and the cleaning with *Calendula essence* is *Arnica/Echinacea comp. powder*, which should be applied to the affected areas and then covered by a dressing: this helps the healing over, dries the lesions and stops them burning. If treated promptly, the infection does not cause harm and responds well to the simple treatment that I have indicated: the lesions regress and are reversible.

In the case of an unrecognized illness and when the lesions are extensive, you should not delay consulting a doctor and then following the prescribed treatment and hygiene measures to avoid complications that could ruin the holiday.

As I have already said, common sense is the best weapon for tackling problems of health.

Shingles: *Herpes zoster*

Shingles, the "holy fire", or "St. Anthony's fire" is caused by a virus (*Herpes varicella zoster*) which is at the origin of both varicella (chicken pox) and *Herpes zoster* (shingles). Varicella is the primary infection, while *Herpes zoster* corresponds to a recurrence, related to reactivation of the virus. It is an important condition on which we would like to reflect briefly and give some practical indications which we consider very useful[81].

Varicella is a childhood disease, which tends to be harmless and heals spontaneously. It needs only rest and a light diet, but its resolution can be helped by the classical remedies for the treatment of inflammation, such as *Apis/Belladonna globules* and possibly *Rhus toxicodendron D6 drops*, alternated every two hours. In adults, however, it is a more serious condition that can give rise to severe consequences requiring medical treatment.

Herpes zoster, commonly known as shingles or, in some countries, as *St. Anthony's fire,* is a neurocutaneous condition characterized by inflammation of a nerve (*ganglioneuritis*) and is associated with a cutaneous eruption along the pathway of a sensory nerve. The disorder starts with a rather intense, dull, poorly localised pain. After three or four days, red blotches appear on the skin, usually arranged along the pathway of a single nerve; soon the blisters that appear transform into pustules that can contain blood. If the patient is elderly or very ill, *Herpes zoster* can cause severe lesions (necrotic), appear gangrenous and be accompanied by intense pain. Shingles occurs most frequently in the regions between the ribs, causing chest pain on only one side of the body:

---

[81] The term "St. Anthony's fire" is still used in various northern European countries to mean ergotism, a common condition in the Middle Ages among the poor who ate rye bread, often infested with a fungal parasite (ergot). This terrible condition, which is much more serious than *Herpes zoster*, is manifested by convulsions, hallucinations or even gangrene. In this chapter "St. Anthony's fire" refers only to *Herpes zoster*, which causes some symptoms resembling the effects of ergot poisoning.

the pain is usually acute and worse during the night. This type of neurological pain is almost always minimal in children and young people, but can be very substantial in the elderly and associated with decreased local sensitivity or even complete loss of sensation, with vasomotor disorders and sweating. The skin lesions heal within two to four weeks and often leave scars so the diagnosis can also be made retrospectively. The disorder may also manifest higher up in the body, in the head, in the region of the *trigeminal nerve*, although it often only affects one of the branches of this nerve. Depending on which of the branches is affected, there may be ocular, lingual, oral or auricular complications. Sometimes the facial nerve may also be affected. The most frequent complications are *neurological:* these can lead to paralysis and chronic effects. Shingles is an important condition and the pain can be continuous, very intense or even intolerable and may have serious consequences, above all in patients over sixty years old who suffer from *Herpes zoster* ophthalmicus (zoster of the eye), which often leaves permanent damage.

We wanted to describe the clinical picture caused by this virus because it should not be underestimated, as often occurs, given that it is not painful in the initial stage of the skin manifestations; however, it does require urgent medical treatment.

Useful practical advice

We anthroposophic doctors have strongly positive experience with regards to pain control in *Herpes zoster,* and above all in the feared complications of post-herpetic neuralgia. One very important treatment is the administration of a purge in the evening; *Epsom salts* (a tablespoon or a sachet in a glass of water), followed in the morning by an *enema* of two litres for adults, are excellent. This treatment activates the largest organ of the immune system: the intestine. Furthermore, since this is a centrifugal illness that tends to move upwards, we use what is called a diverting *therapy*, that is, we invert, at least in part, the direction of the inflammatory wave through gentle irritation and stimulation of the intestinal system. This safe and effective treatment notably reduces both the severity of the disorder and the risk of complications and should be associated for at least ten days with a "light diet" with a low content of protein and salt, for example, boiled rice or oatmeal cooked in water and dressed with only oil, organic rice or spelt biscuits, bitter green vegetables together with carrots, courgettes, beetroot, lettuce (all vegetables must be only boiled and then dressed with olive oil), cooked fruit, squeezed fruit juices, blended fruit and vegetables, such as the classical carrot-apple combination with a bit of beetroot, and barley coffee.

A reflection
Art in treatment. The work of a doctor can become a therapeutic fine-tuning if you help him to aspire to the care of the *"ignis sacer"*, the "holy fire". We anthroposophic doctors have a special fondness for the work of the great artist Grünewald who, in his masterpiece *The Isenheim Altarpiece*[82], immortalised two saints: St. Anthony and St. Sebastian, healers of the sick. It is St. Anthony who is indicated as the healer of "St. Anthony's fire", as shown by the presence of a patient with the "holy fire" among the devilish monsters that attack the saint from all directions.

---

82 *The Isenheim Altarpiece* by Grünewald is displayed in the Alsatian city of Colmar in France, and is one of the classical visits for students of the anthroposophic medical courses, particularly for those taking place in Dornach/Arlesheim, given the proximity of Colmar to Basel. Dear readers, I do encourage you to go and see this painting: it really is a profoundly stirring experience.

Cold sores: *Herpes simplex*

Herpes simplex infection is very common. Its clinical manifestations on the skin and mucosal membranes, popularly called *cold sores* or *febrile blisters*, tend to alternate with latent periods and then re-appear. The lesions that affect the upper part of the body, particularly the face and mucosa of the oral cavity (labial herpes) are related to a virus, *Herpes simplex* type 1, while the lesions involving the genital area and surrounding skin (genital herpes) are caused by *Herpes simplex* virus type 2; this latter type of virus is also responsible for neonatal herpes, an infection caused by contagion of the neonate during delivery. The diagnosis is simple in adults, because the clinical appearance of the lesions is easy to recognize. The diagnosis in children is relatively more difficult because labial herpes can be confused with impetigo. Although it is true that the virus is originally transmitted from herpetic lesions by direct interpersonal contact, through the saliva in healthy carriers or through sexual activity for genital herpes, anthroposophic medicine disagrees strongly with the use of typical local treatments with antiviral drugs that suppress the manifestations of the illness and tend to make it become chronic. How often do we examine patients who are having ever more frequent attacks, reaching the point at which the illness is almost continuously present?

According to some authors, almost the entire adult population are carriers of the herpes virus in a latent state and are, therefore, potentially at risk of recurrences; however, epidemiological studies indicate that the recurrence rate is about 10%. This implies that we must work to strengthen the body's defences, taking into account that the molecular mechanisms underlying the establishment and maintenance of the latent state, and also the reactivations, have not yet been clarified despite being the object of extensive investigation. Understanding these mechanisms will be important in the battle to defeat this virus as part of the management of recurrent infections. Anthroposophic medicine is aimed at strengthening the spontaneous defences of the body against those triggering factors that, by transiently weakening cellular defences that control the virus, enable reactivation of the herpes infection. We are interested in research that has implicated general infections, overtiredness, cold, exposure to strong sunlight, menstruation, sexual intercourse, stress, some drugs and, finally, some foods. For example, particular attention is currently being given to the diet, even if a relationship between food eaten and the circumscribed, recurrent forms of herpes has never been the focus of controlled clinical trials. Recently, conventional medicine has identified some foods that should be eliminated from the diet of people who suffer frequently from labial herpes and some which, on the other hand, could prevent recurrences. One possible culprit for the reactivation of the latent virus is *arginine*, an amino acid that is a component of proteins and necessary for viral replication. It is, therefore, worthwhile checking the labels of pre-packed food to ensure that this amino acid is not contained in the food. Furthermore, athletes should check that it is not contained in any supplements that they may take during their training. Foods that are rich in this amino acid should be banned, particularly walnuts, almonds, peanuts, chocolate and some types of red wine, but also fatty foods, very spicy foods and foods based on gelatine. High doses of vitamin C can trigger an acute herpes attack, as can all food that induce allergies or intolerance. Coconut, wheat, corn, and Brussels sprouts are all possible risk factors. I have given this information to show that these recommendations are similar to those that an anthroposophic doctor gives on the basis of a conception of illness as a problem of a person as a whole: a skin disorder leads us spontaneously to choose foods that rebalance the nerve-sense pole, thus foods rich in mineral salts, such as vegetable roots, and to reduce the intake of foods containing a large amount of "convenient", but dangerous proteins. We are not convinced by the restrictive idea that a single amino acid is responsible for an illness, because this contrasts with the clinical experience of conventional medicine itself, which has already identified another amino acid, *lysine*, that plays a protective role, antagonising the metabolic effect of arginine: if lysine prevails over arginine, the synthesis of arginine-rich proteins necessary for viral replication is blocked.

Effectively, by administering high doses of lysine, we do hamper recurrences of cold sores. This is not, however, a cure since when the lysine supplementation is stopped, the herpes recurs within one to four weeks.

We risk getting sucked into a game of numbers, which is not easy to follow: indeed, the advised lysine supplementation (at least two grams a day) seems to be implicated in raising cholesterol levels in the blood. Furthermore, arginine is essential for stimulating the production of growth hormone and it would, therefore, certainly be an error to counteract its presence in growing individuals, such as children, although these are often affected by *Herpes simplex*. Besides, growth hormone has useful functions throughout life, not only in infancy and adolescence. We have already criticised one-sided thinking and the obvious commercial interests behind the exaggerated use of integrators and dietary supplements, often sold as non-conventional medicines, but in reality the expression of extremely mechanistic thoughts and with strongly contradictory results.

Large amounts of lysine are found in fish, meat, but also milk,, cheese and, above all, in legumes such as chickpeas and peas, which usually form a substantial part of natural diets. The seeds of amaranth, a spectacular plant with clusters of reddish purple flowers, formed the basis of the diet of the Inca and Aztec civilisations. These civilisations attributed miraculous powers to amaranth seeds and worshipped the plant as a dwelling place of a god. Consumption of this plant, prohibited by the Spanish conquistadors, has now been resumed in natural diets: since these seeds are very rich in lysine, they combine well with the cereals of our tradition. For example, amaranth flakes can be used together with oatmeal in muesli in the morning or in vegetable soup in the evening. The anthroposophic approach concerns a broader front: trying to learn good dietary habits and a healthy lifestyle in which the body finds a balance not only between the amino acids present in food, but also in daily conduct. We know that the virus often erupts after a sleepless night or after having eaten very spicy food or after excessive exposure to the sun. This should teach us something. I really feel that I can say that our clinical experience is very positive: with our treatments, herpes disappears completely or manifests itself only very rarely.

We have a series of natural remedies in homeopathic doses against herpes, including *Rhus toxicodendron*, *Ranunculus bulbosus*, *Mezereum*, *Cantharis*, and *Graphites*, which are a precious opportunity if prescribed appropriately on the basis of the individual clinical picture. The proper treatment of recurrent herpes, chronically suppressed by local allopathic remedies, often passes through a very violent and obvious eruption which must be left to burn out. I warn patients of this worsening, even though I can never find the right words to prevent the complaints and grievances: a face disfigured, even if only temporarily, during treatment is not easy to accept. However, once the critical phase has passed, the absence of recurrences generates reciprocal satisfaction and strengthens the doctor-patient relationship. A treatment involving the whole person promotes the action of the immune system in its entirety and frees the person from the constant thoughts of being infected or having infected someone. Seasonal recurrences can be prevented by using, for example, a *lip-stick with a sunscreen* from the earliest exposure to sun in the spring and not staying in the sun during the hottest hours of the day, when the sun's rays are most dangerous.

The authoritative American medical journal, "JAMA" estimated that there are fifty million Americans infected by genital herpes. Less than 10% of these people know that they carry the infection, because the virus often gives no trouble, and asymptomatic carriers therefore become "vehicles" that spread the infection. The virus may remain latent for a long time and the illness can also be transmitted within a monogamous couple because the first contagion may have occurred during a previous relationship a very long time ago. We need a medicine of human dimensions that accepts that being ill is part of the human condition and that our task is not to learn to recognize the very earliest symptoms of herpes, but rather to lead a life worth living: sometimes this is less difficult and more enjoyable than constantly trying to escape the human condition by vaccinating against every possible problem or, worse still, rejecting carriers of the virus.

If, perhaps, the herpes reappears after years, this should be seen as a precious warning, almost as if a slightly invasive "friend" wants to make us understand that we are exaggerating in something. It warns us that we must once again question ourselves and admit honestly that we have abandoned our good habits, often falling into the trap of the "strains and stresses of modern life", as the great actor Ernesto Calindri said in the famous advertisement for an Italian bitter made of artichokes that he sipped while sitting in the middle of city traffic whizzing by on either side. Consult your anthroposophic doctor for the treatment of this small manifestation of herpes which punctuates our hectic life, in order to obtain a therapy that is a process of personal growth and inner dialogue.

As a symptomatic treatment for local manifestations of the infection, I advise *Calendula essence 20%*. This can be dabbed undiluted on lesions at the start of the eruptions. Once the blisters have formed, we can use 10 or 15 drops of the essence in a tablespoon of water to make compresses; in the florid state we can also use *Calendula 10% ointment,* applied locally a couple of times a day.

Warts: an unpleasant manifestation

Warts are growths of viral origin which present as flat or raised papulous excrescences on the skin. Common warts (verruca vulgaris) are fairly frequent and occur on the back of the hands, the fingers, legs and feet. One fascinating aspect of these growths is that they have a different appearance depending on where they develop on the body, which is simply one more proof that man is a microcosm: just as a plant changes shape according to the habitat in which it grows, so warts differ depending on the body surface. This shows that the viral origin of the problem does not explain the whole phenomenon. How many times have I been told: "I caught a verruca at the swimming pool because I didn't have my flip-flops".
I personally know swimming teachers who have not worn flip-flops for years and have never caught a verruca! Another interesting point is the vegetative aspect: a wart is like a mushroom that grows on the skin; even in medical language the term vegetation is used to described warty growths. Here we have a key to the diagnosis, which comes directly from the observation: warts are related to the ether body, to the vital body that grows and tends to assume an oval shape.
What constrains and holds back the ether body from its tendency to vegetate, to grow constantly, and make each one of us an "egg"? It is the astral body that has the task of holding, containing and giving form to the etheric growth; a wart is a sort of "stretch mark" in the astral network which envelops the ether at the periphery of the body.
We can take account of this aspect in treatment and "dream" an elegant, refined cure, as a song interpreted by a great singer modifies our astral body, transmitting emotions to us; and what are emotions? They are manifestations of the astral body, and would it not, therefore, be wonderful to respond to an unpleasant manifestation with the profoundly human voice of Aretha Franklin, the queen of soul? Soul, the musical genre, just as our soul? And

is the soul not the astral body? The great German poet Novalis said: *"you cannot pick a flower without disturbing a star"*, and referred to the emotionally stirring interconnection that crosses the entire universe.

Indeed, precisely the "humble" wart, a disorder snubbed by medicine, can become fascinating for the very noble possibility that it offers us to treat the human being as a microcosm: if we put a drop of medicine onto the tongue of a patient, just a drop at a homeopathic dose (that is, without the presence of specific molecules of the substance detectable by chemical analyses), a tiny "light" descends into the depths of the body and far, far away, at a sidereal distance, a small smile appears, a fine breeze that "pushes" the wart and brings the etheric forces back to their place. I believe that this is poetry, poetry in healing.

The patients, with the pragmatism typical of the current age, note only that the wart has disappeared, perhaps giving more value to other aspects of the treatment, but for the doctor it is an important victory.

Indeed, a great poet and dermatologist, Gottfried Benn, wrote[83]: *"A voice and the warts fall, so warts, studied in a hundred ways under a microscope, disappear as a result of persuasion. Small cancers, caused by a live virus, wither through the effect of an energetic word. It is clear that the human being is something different from what my science teaches me, he is not such a lowly, dense thing, he is not a thing whose carcass must be treated with gas tubes and rubber piping in order to be healed and to investigate its nature"*.

Everyone knows that warts are treated by folk healers with "gestures". Instead of playing the outraged moralist, it is worth trying to understand how we can act on the astral body in a positive and ethically correct way, respecting the patient's freedom. This freedom is the condition that an anthroposophic doctor and a conscious patient both want to be fully respected.

---

[83] Gottfried Benn, Probleme der Lyrik, Klett-Cotta Verlag (German ed.), 2011.

Some simple advice

Warts can be "persuaded" by the latex, the sap-like fluid of plants; anthroposophic medicine teaches us that a curative principle, called the "plastic-dynamic system", develops in the latex of plants, a force capable of maintaining life, which is something "sticky". I know what some of you are thinking and you are right: the greatest need to maintain life is in the genital fluids. The anthroposophic remedies try to implement this principle every time that a curative substance needs to be helped in its effect on an organ or a function; the plant, in its infinite wisdom, does this spontaneously.

For example, many people know that the yellowish-orange latex of *chelidonium* (the greater celandine), which oozes out when the leaves are detached from the plant, is an excellent treatment for resolving warts[84]. In South American countries the latex of *papaya* is used to treat warts and eczema. The latex of the leaves of the *fig* plays the same role, as does that of *poinsettia* (Christmas star). A useful remedy that combines *garlic*[85], the "stinking rose", and various essential oils (oregano, thyme, thuja, rosemary, niaouli, etc.) is the *Herbal wart cream* (*Crema all'Erba Porraia*), which is applied locally. The wart must be kept covered with the cream for some weeks in order to obtain a positive effect. A use-

---

[84] I remember with nostalgia my dear anthroposophic colleagues, Roberto Meda and Patrizia Garavelli, and the small wild garden of their clinic, where I worked for many years. Every year, the greater celandine grew spontaneously in the garden and we respected its presence. I also remember a patient who lived nearby and who, on my advice, came to get a leaf of celandine a day for a long time until the wart he had surrendered and left him. I owe this patient the recommendation to read the book by Benn.

[85] Garlic is a formidable remedy; I remember that back in the nineteen-seventies, together with the biologist Giuseppe Ferraro, who subsequently created the herbal wart remedy, we were using it for warts with excellent results. Through studying the problem, we discovered that a bulb of garlic contains an exceptional "plastic-dynamic system" and has at least a dual action: on the one hand it is has potent antiviral, antibacterial, antifungal and anti-parasitic properties, but on the other hand it is an excellent immuno-stimulant as well as a "de-keratiniser", since it is able to remove hard dead skin, an action that is exploited in the treatment of callouses and warts.

ful remedy is *Thuja occidentalis 10% ointment*: after having washed the wart with hot water, the ointment is applied locally and covered with a piece of plaster tape. When the warts are on the feet or legs, apply the ointment once or twice a day, changing the plaster each time; when the warts are on the hands, the ointment should be applied several times a day. I recommend perseverance because the effect usually begins after at least one or two months. We can strengthen this treatment with *Thuja ointment* and give an oral treatment, *Thuja D6*, 10 drops in a little water, before the three meals; persevere with the treatment for at least two months.

Warts, vaccinations and the immune system
In susceptible subjects, warts characteristically appear after a vaccination, a clear sign of weakened defences. If this happens to you, tell your anthroposophic doctor and get advice on how to treat yourself after every vaccination; in general, my advice is only to have the obligatory vaccinations.

It is important to precede surgical removal of warts by an internal treatment that enables the immune system to control or at least to stop the growth and spread of the warts. This way of proceeding, telling your doctor that you have warts and taking appropriate anthroposophic treatment, reduces the risk of recurrences and spread which are very common after surgery.

One proof of what I have said is that the spread of numerous warts is typical of diseases in which there is a state of immunosuppression, such as AIDS and Hodgkin's lymphoma, or after chemotherapy.

Acne and boils

Acne
Acne is a complex disorder related to hormonal factors, as shown by its typical onset in puberty, but it is also related to a weakness in the metabolism and in particular in the liver and intestinal system. The local proliferation of bacteria in the skin eruption is only the final aspect of a complex process that starts from the innermost part of the body.

Attention to the diet
Despite what everyone says, *diet* is very important in acne; eruption means "to break out": what breaks out is what the forces of the metabolism can no longer control. In severe cases we advise a week of a diet based on raw biodynamic, or at least organic, food, in particular fruit and coloured vegetables such as carrots, beetroot and red cabbage salad.
This should be followed by four weeks of a vegetarian diet based on well-cooked, biodynamic wholemeal cereals, organic whole grain bread, carrots, beetroots, seasonal vegetables, a little yoghurt (not cold), cottage cheese made from sheep's milk, sour milk, seasonal fruits cooked without sugar, barley coffee or drinks made from other organic cereals and large amounts of water. Meat, fish or pulses can then be added, according to personal taste, three times a week.
Food that should not be eaten includes pork, beef, all types of cured meats, smoked foods, products based on refined wheat and, in general, white flour (Kamut wheat flour is allowed), sugar-based food, milk and dairy products, fermented cheeses, eggs as such (food containing eggs is permitted), processed and conserved foods, such as vegetables in brine, wine and alcohol in any form, including beer.
One important recommendation is to chew food carefully to improve the region of the metabolism. Thorough chewing is the equivalent of psychosomatic treatment for the metabolic sphere,

which is shaken by the tensions and frustrations of adolescence, the typical age of onset of this disorder.

Hygienic measures
For facial cleansing and local remedies, I recommend consulting an aesthetician who uses the Hauschka method; this method gives really excellent results and respects the skin.
A good starting product for facial cleansing is simply *Iris milk cleanser*; to apply with cotton balls, just as any ordinary cleanser, after having rinsed the face with very hot water. This can be alternated with a *purifying lotion* (*Aknedoron*), to use three times a week for a greater draining effect.
A useful treatment is a weekly application of a *face mask of fine green clay,* made of the following constituents:
fine green clay, one glass;
honey, one teaspoon;
extra virgin oil of organic olives or sweet almonds, one teaspoon; still mineral water, half a glass.
Dissolve the honey in the glass of water and then add the oil, mixing everything together well; then, stirring continuously, gradually add the glass of green clay. Continue to mix energetically until obtaining a smooth, glossy cream. At this point you could add a spoonful of fresh lemon juice, continuing to mix well.
Using a spatula, apply the mask to the face and forehead, leave in place for ten minutes and then remove it, using a sponge moistened with warm water. The skin will become softer and less oily and the acne lesions will heal more quickly.
Calendula essence, one part diluted in ten parts of warm water, for wet compresses on the affected areas; this is always useful to draw the spots and for disinfection.
Ointments are not usually helpful and may even be counterproductive.
Your anthroposophic doctor can help you with treatment that acts very deeply within the body, rebalancing the hormonal sphere and supporting the metabolism; you must, however, be patient.

Boils, impetigo and skin abscesses

These are well-known and very frequent infections of the skin due to contamination of very small traumatic or non-traumatic lesions by bacteria normally present on the skin or on the object that has caused the trauma; otherwise they are related to obstruction of the hair bulb. The same dietary rules indicated for acne also apply in cases of widespread and recurrent furuncles. The main infections of this type are impetigo and skin abscesses.

Impetigo is a skin infection characterized by groups of vesicles, pustules or blisters which tend to form scabs (see the chapter on impetigo).

Skin abscesses occur in the deep layers of the skin and are caused by infections of sebaceous glands or obstruction of the hair follicles with accumulation of pus. The classical furuncle (boil) forms at the bottom of the hair bulb. If it forms around the nail it is called a *whitlow*.

The treatment involves very hot compresses with *Calendula essence*; dilute one part of *Calendula* in ten parts of hot water. If there are general symptoms, such as fever, use *Apis/Belladonna globules*: the dose for children is 5-7 globules every two hours, that for adults is 10 globules. Alternate every hour this remedy with *Lachesis comp. globules*, particularly in cases of impetigo. Impetigo is a typical complication of scratching in atopic eczema and also frequently affects children in the summer, because their exposed skin is made weaker by the sun and becomes more susceptible to infections. Repeated micro-lesions, scratching the skin with dirty fingers and insect bites, even simple mosquito bites, can all contribute to the development of impetigo.

An excellent treatment for classic furuncles and isolated skin abscesses is a *poultice of fine green clay*.

Subsequently use *Mercurialis comp. ointment* which can also be applied with a dressing; this is excellent for whitlows, too. However, my favourite treatment for a whitlow remains that of sticking the affected finger into a cherry tomato and then bandaging it, changing the dressing every day until the whitlow is healed; this is very effective and children think that it is fun.

In the case of large skin abscesses, an internal treatment should be tried. Such treatment is:
Apis D3 drops,
Belladonna D4 drops,
5-7 drops of both remedies in a little water, alternated every hour with:
Myristica sebifera comp. globules, 10 globules to dissolve in the mouth.
The doses should be halved for children.
An application of *Ichthammol ointment* can be useful to mature the lesions and draw out the pus; the lesion can then be disinfected with diluted *Calendula essence* and treated with *Mercurialis comp.*
Myristica sebifera ointment, which is considered a sort of "scalpel" of homeopathic medicine because it helps even deep abscesses come to a head.
In the more severe cases and those that do not heal, your doctor may consider that a boil needs to be lanced.

Eczema and dermatitis

Eczema: the skin becomes nerve
Here we are talking about the so-called constitutional eczema, atopic eczema or atopic dermatitis. In German this disorder is called *"Neurodermitis"*, indicating a skin disorder that, for psychosomatic reasons or certain psychological factors, induces the individual to scratch his skin. From our point of view this illness highlights the skin's tendency to become conscious activity, to "become nerve", showing the relationship, mediated by the immune system, between the nervous system and skin disorders. Modern immunology provides an excellent opportunity to bring the anthropological and physiological concepts of anthroposophic medicine closer together.
Atopic dermatitis is an inflammatory disorder that tends to recur and become chronic. It is particularly common among small children, affecting about 10% of such children. Here we are in the field of allergic conditions, such as asthma and allergic rhinitis, so I refer the reader to the chapters on these subjects; all these conditions are essentially a single disorder with varied manifestations.
Dermatitis is the expression, on a genetic background, of a tendency to produce antibodies to substances (allergens) that are not real enemies. If this response occurs in the skin, the subject develops dermatitis: the skin is dry, rough and "delicate", with a tendency to inflammation and itching.
Given the chronic nature of the disorder, this skin condition can be very challenging from the point of view of the soul, both for the child and for his parents. Some environmental and dietary factors are very important in its onset, such as cow's milk, egg white, walnuts, soy flour and wheat gluten. Pollen, the fur and dander of some animals (for example, cats, dogs and horses) and dust mites also play an important role in worsening or triggering eczema. Some textile fibres such as wool, but also synthetic fibres, can exacerbate the itching.

A marine environment almost always has a positive effect.

The lesions are reddened, often scaly and very itchy; the liquid that oozes out worsens the lesions. The distress is caused by the itching and the vicious cycle that it sets up: itching, which causes scratch lesions which, in turn, cause intense itching and worsen the inflammation.

In early infancy, the eruptions are most common on the face and scalp; subsequently they can develop in the large skin creases of the back of the knees, the wrists, inner elbows and at the joints of the hands.

The skin of affected children is unable to produce adequate amounts of lipids (to form a hydrolipid covering), and so it is helpful to apply oily ointments at least once a day.

One basic ointment is *Dulcamara/Lysimachia ointment*, which has a healing effect and can be associated with an oilier ointment such as *Unguentum rosatum, Biolenil, Halicar* ointment. *Allergel A.S.* has the effect of soothing the itching.

Treatment with herbal baths can also be useful: one excellent combination is an *anti-eczema tea* made from equal amounts of *elderberry flower / nettle leaves / heart's ease flowers / chamomile flowers / juniper flowers*. Care must be given to the quality of the constituents, which should be at least organic, but preferably biodynamic.

Pour a teaspoonful into a cup of boiling water and leave to rest, covered, for ten minutes before filtering and adding to the water in a bath; use hot water although taking care not to scald yourself. This tea can also be used for local compresses; apply a piece of cotton soaked in the tea to the affected area and cover in order to keep in the warmth.

The treatment of eczema inevitably requires the help of a doctor. I limit myself here to mentioning only the "typical" anthroposophic remedy for skin conditions: *Lysimachia/Solanum Dulcamara drops*, 10 drops before the three meals for adults, 5 drops for children. This remedy harmonises growth processes in such a way that the "I" can enter the power of light of the silica that helps the human being rediscover a new boundary with the world. It takes a long time to work, but it helps to find the way again in a condition that is much influenced by contemporary lifestyle.

I recommend avoiding the use of cortisone creams as much as possible; these are a real temptation, but make the illness descend into the body predisposing the subject to asthma in the years to come. Asthma is more difficult to treat than eczema, which tends to resolve spontaneously or become less severe with growth. At last, conventional medicine is supporting this point of view, which we anthroposophists have been putting forward for many years[86].

I believe that conventional medicine is correct when it criticises some doctors of complementary medicine who prescribe cortisone together with various homeopathic treatments and herbal remedies without informing the patients of what they are receiving.

Dietary indications are particularly important in the treatment of eczema. Good prevention is based on prolonged, complete breastfeeding, followed by a very slow introduction of new foods into the diet over the course of the first two years of life. Furthermore, it is important to limit the intake of sugar and proteins; dairy products can facilitate the development of allergic rashes. Yoghurt, however, is often well tolerated and can be eaten in the morning with muesli or cereals, although cold yoghurt directly from the fridge is to be avoided. I advise that you take what you want to eat at breakfast the next morning out the refrigerator before going to bed. Once again, I repeat that the three foods with the highest risk are milk, eggs and walnuts. Seasonal fruits and vegetables, dressed with olive oil, are very important.

With satisfaction, I prescribe essential fatty acids to be taken by

---

86 "In most cases the most effective treatment for atopic dermatitis is topical, i.e. applied to the skin. However, care must be taken not to abuse the use of corticosteroids. Moisturisers should be used constantly. This is a treatment trend that is gaining hold throughout Europe" (Dr. Carlo Gelmetti, Dr. Serena Speic, Institute of Dermatological Sciences, University of Milan, Italy).

mouth. Although these fatty acids, such as linoleic acid, are contained in *borage oil* and *evening primrose oil,* for example, it is still worth trusting the advice of your doctor for products of known quality. Essential fatty acids are recommended because they are necessary for the correct structure of the cell membrane and because they are the metabolic precursors of substances that maintain the normal impermeability of the skin to water and other liquids. They are also involved in the transport and metabolism of cholesterol.

Care should be taken to rinse underwear very thoroughly to avoid residues of detergents. It is better not to use fabric softeners; they can be replaced by some vinegar, added to the last rinse, as our grandmothers well knew.

Contact dermatitis

In adults, the similarity between the symptoms of atopic dermatitis and contact dermatitis can create some confusion at the time of diagnosis. Both are characterized by altered barrier function, thickening, dryness and itching of the skin. They do, however, differ with regards to a genetic predisposition and the consequent immune response, which is immediate in atopic dermatitis and delayed in contact dermatitis.

An allergic contact dermatitis, caused as we have said, by delayed hypersensitivity, may create problems in subjects with an atopic constitution as well as in non-atopic individuals. Although the signs and symptoms are very similar between the two forms, and both have a genetic background, immunologically the two hypersensitivity reactions are different.

In most cases of atopic dermatitis the substances causing the allergic reaction (antigens) are proteins, whereas in contact dermatitis the triggering molecules (haptens) may be very small (with a much lower molecular weight) and must combine with proteins to become "allergising" (complete antigens).

Unfortunately, numerous substances can cause contact eczema. Here I shall discuss just one, which is very widespread in our society: *nickel sulphate*. This is present in chromium-plated objects, but also in photocopies, keys and, unfortunately, also in the coins of some countries, for example the coins of one and two euros, which contain enough nickel to cause contact eczema in people allergic to this metal, with consequent inflammation of the skin or the appearance of the irritating blisters. Here it is not alternative medicine that is in question, and yet we doctors have not been listened to, even about the introduction of coins that are really harmful to many patients.

Piercing, which is increasingly fashionable among the young, can be a cause of eczema. We should at least try to advise "nickel-free" piercing.

A person with dermatitis should always have an evaluation of possible allergies; "patch tests", in particular, can identify the cause of a contact dermatitis.

Depending on the causative agent, certain lifestyle indications can be given; for example, nickel sulphate is found in numerous metal objects used in the household (scissors, kitchen utensils, the sink, etc.), in the medical, surgical and dental professions, in clothing (jewelry, buttons, buckles, belts, earrings), as well as in coins, handles, chairs, etc. Contact with these objects and, in general, with nickel-containing metals, as well as with cement, washing powder, and hair dyes, must be avoided; enamelled pans, pyrex or terracotta utensils are advised for cooking. Some dietary precautions should also be taken; in fact, trace amounts of nickel are present in many types of food which should, therefore, be avoided; examples are tinned food, herrings, oysters, asparagus, lentils, beans, peas, lettuce, cabbage, tomatoes, hazel nuts and liquorice.

Besides the measures described above, a good tea is useful for adults with eczema.

Decoction of elm bark: this is rich in bitter substances with anti-inflammatory properties and had astringent effect due to the presence of tannins. Pour three tablespoons of elm bark into a litre and a half of water, boil for ten minutes and then filter. Drink two or three cups of the warmed decoction each day. Store in a refrigerator for a couple of days, but no more.

Palpebral eczema

Nickel is a substance often present in mascara, eye-shadows and eye-pencils, and can, therefore cause palpebral eczema in subjects sensitive to this metal. Furthermore, it has been shown that in sensitive people, even particles of nickel transferred to the eyelids by the hands can cause eczema. For example, some cases of palpebral dermatitis have been resolved by banning the use of metal nail-files. The same indications made for contact dermatitis also apply to palpebral eczema.

Mycoses: fungi on the skin

Mycoses are ever more frequent infections of the skin caused by micro-organisms (yeasts or fungi) which must be attached to another organism in order to survive. These micro-organisms prefer warm, humid environments and, therefore, they readily flourish in the warmer areas of the body, such as the groin, armpits and between the toes. The most frequent forms are *pityriasis (or tinea) versicolor, ringworm* and *candidiasis (thrush)*.

Pityriasis versicolor is caused by *Pityrosporum orbiculare*. It localises in greasy areas of the skin, such as the back, head, arms and the upper part of the chest where the warmth and abundant sweating promote its growth. The characteristic white, roundish, well-defined lesions, covered with small scales like dandruff, then appear.

Ringworm is caused by other types of fungi, particularly those of the genus *Trichophyton*. The lesions are yellowish and scaly, with fissures, reddening, itching and pain.

Candidiasis, caused by fungi of the genus *Candida*, develops in conditions of immune system impairment. It can become established in the mouth (stomatitis, thrush), in skin folds, particularly below the breasts in obese women (intertrigo), between the toes and at the edges of the nails. The vaginal form, usually detected by a gynaecologist, is characteristic.

Classical medicine uses *antifungal drugs* applied locally or taken orally.

Unfortunately, what is lacking is an overall view appreciating that this illness is not just a local infection to be resolved with creams or vaginal ovules or pessaries. It should be considered a strange superstition to state the people who go to swimming pools are more susceptible to fungal infections of the toes (athlete's foot); in fact, there are numerous swimming teachers who have never had a fungal infection. As we have been teaching for years, this is a problem involving the intestinal immune system and its capacity to control the proliferation of fungi; we do, therefore, believe that the strategy is not that of the usual antifungal treatments with a palliative effect, but that of working on the intestine, because this is very probably the centre of the immune imbalance that has opened up the way to the infection.

I draw particular satisfaction from saying that modern immunology has reached the same conclusions long since proposed by anthroposophic medicine in its global vision of the human being. If "plants" grow on my skin, it means that the ether body is imbalanced at the boundaries of the body; our fundamental boundaries, our periphery, have the intestine at the centre and the skin at the exterior. The silica process works to give substrate to the "I", to make our boundaries operative both within the intestine and at the exterior on the skin; thus antifungal drugs are not sufficient for the treatment of these disorders which often require a general rebalancing of the silica metabolism, we must act on lifestyle.

I repeat, once more, that there is no such thing as a local disease: succeeding in improving or curing a recurrent fungal infection through the use of diet of biodynamic wholemeal cereals is also a profound personal satisfaction, recovering one's own identity and human dimension.

Here is one small tip before the real treatment:

Calendula essence, this is useful for some small fungal lesions. Dilute one part of *Calendula* in ten parts of warm water, moisten some gauze with the solution obtained and apply the compress to the affected area for ten minutes in the morning and again in the evening.

Cuprum 0.4% / Tabacum D6 ointment; apply after the compress.

Fungal infections of the feet and toes (athlete's foot)

I recommend very hot foot baths with an *anti-eczema tea*[87]. After having dried the feet, sprinkle them with *Arnica/Echinacea comp. powder.*

Calluses

I would like to emphasize that calluses derive from a poor posture, for example, a defect in the spinal column increases the load and stress on one part of the foot which reacts to the continuous pressure with an increase in the thickness of the skin; this also occurs as the consequence of the ever more frequent use of inappropriate shoes, such as those that are too pointed or have heels that are too high.

One little tip for reddened calluses is to apply a small gauze moistened with *Calendula essence* to the callus once a day and cover it with a plaster; this remedy relieves the inflammation and reduces the callosity.

Organic raisins: apply half of a raisin cut in two and bandage it to the callus. Remove the raisin after 24 hours and repeat the procedure for the next three to four days. Then remove the callus with tweezers.

Some practical advice

One extremely common mistake is to wear shoes that are too short, which subject the feet to a constant state of constriction. Do not trust the number of the shoe size, but try the shoes on before buying them; the ideal is about half a size larger.

The extremely expensive trainers that youngsters wear are almost always harmful to the back because they are technical shoes designed for a specific function such as running and do not, perhaps, absorb the stresses of normal walking in our unyielding world of asphalt and cement. In childhood the foot is still malleable, containing cartilage, and tends to change shape depending

---

[87] The tea is described in the first section of this chapter.

on the stimuli it receives: it is for this reason that the feet of our youngsters are so flat and shapeless.
Sporting activities constitute only a small part of our everyday life. Leather shoes are still the ideal for allowing the feet to breathe and for softening the impact with our inelastic world.

Chilblains

Chilblains are lesions due to the cold which manifest, in susceptible individuals, as a painful swelling of the parts of the body most exposed to cold (fingers, toes, heels and ears). The cause is an alteration in the venous circulation of the peripheral part of the body affected. Prevention consists in adequate protection from the cold with socks, gloves, ear muffs and comfortable shoes. Chilblains are also known as "erythema pernio".

A *decoction of oak bark* has always given good results in the treatment of chilblains. This decoction is prepared by pouring 2 to 3 cooking spoons of oak bark into a litre of cold water, bringing to boil and boiling for five minutes. Immerge the hands or feet into the filtered liquid. The recommended temperature for the hand or foot bath, which should last 10-20 minutes, is about 40°C.

Bites and stings

On this subject I only want to give a few tips, appealing to common sense and general knowledge of first aid, which goes beyond the scope of this book.

Animal bites
Calendula essence dilution, for external use. All animal bites (by cats, dogs, horses, etc.) should be washed immediately with copious amounts of water and then disinfected thoroughly. I recommend *Calendula*: dilute one part (for example, a teaspoonful) in nine parts of water. This solution is used to wash the wound carefully, which should then be covered with gauze soaked with the same solution. The *Calendula* gauze compresses not only disinfect and cure the wound, but also promote good healing. It is worth observing the behaviour of the animal in the days following the bite and should the animal require treatment for any illnesses, report this to the doctor.

A very useful remedy in the case of fright or shock, but also to help the process of wound healing, is *Arnica planta tota D3 drops*, 10 drops every three or four hours for several days; in the case of bigger injuries, change to *Arnica planta tota D6*, 10 drops three times a day, continued for at least seven days.

A doctor must be consulted in the case of bites by rats, snakes, spiders, scorpions or ticks.

Stings by bees, hornets and wasps
Stings by these insects can be a source of intense pain, but also swelling. Besides removing the stinger (if present) with tweezers, trying not to break it, you could also use a poison-aspirating syringe (if not available, even an ordinary syringe without the needle can help to extract the stinger and blood). Dabbing the site of the sting with *ammonia* or undiluted *Calendula* can give a certain benefit, as can applying *ice*. In any case it is then useful to disinfect the area thoroughly with diluted *Calendula*.

Apis mellifica D6 drops or *granules* are very effective if administered immediately after the sting at a dose of 10-15 drops or 3-5 granules. This remedy should always be kept at hand, particularly in the countryside. The remedy should be taken every half hour. High doses are also given to children until the swelling disappears. The remarkable ability of such a diluted remedy, taken by mouth, to control inflammation should remove any doubts about the efficacy of natural medicines and homeopathic powers. I have had the occasion to astonish a medical friend, poorly disposed to natural therapies, by healing his daughter from a large wasp sting.

A sting in the mouth or throat is a much more serious emergency. In these cases it is essential to go to the local Accident and Emergency department immediately, where the appropriate medicines will be prescribed (cortisone, injectable anti-histamines, adrenaline). During the journey to the hospital, you can use ice-cubes which, held in the mouth, cause vasoconstriction thus slowing the development of any obstructive swelling. People who are hypersensitive to bee or wasp stings should also be taken immediately to an Accident and Emergency department if they are stung, because they are at risk of anaphylactic shock. These people should always have cortisone, prescribed by their doctor, at hand so that they can be given an injection immediately after a sting. Any amateurism in matters of health is unforgiveable.

Mosquito bites
Apis mellifica D30 drops. This is an excellent preventive remedy for children, but also for adults, particularly for the ever increasing number of individuals who are hypersensitive to insect bites, especially those of the mosquito. The treatment consists of 10 drops three times a day in a little water for adults and 5 drops, again three times a day, for children. The treatment should be started one or two months before the critical period and continued for at least three months.

This remedy is suited to damping the excessive reactivity caused by pollutants absorbed by the mosquitoes, which make the "dialogue" between the human being and insect so deafening. Indeed, a noble insect such as the bee can restore a confused immune system to that same harmony present in a beehive. This prevention is particularly useful in those children who tend to cause secondary infections of the mosquito bites by scratching the lesions with their nails that are not exactly sterile...

Given that this is a medical treatment, I just mention that this remedy is a fundamental element in reducing the risk of anaphylactic shock in people who have been sensitised to bee or wasp stings, who, out of a perverse law of existence, are stung far more than chance alone would allow: the more they are at risk, the more they are stung! The advice concerning the Accident and Emergency department and cortisone therapy is still valid, but it may be interesting to ask your anthroposophic doctor to prescribe a non-specific desensitising programme such as *Apis*.

Basil: no-one is denied a leaf
Finally, I would like to remind you that an excellent remedy for children stung by mosquitoes is a of leaf of basil applied directly onto the affected site: it reduces the itching and redness. I learnt this remedy from a taxi-driver in Milan, who I take this occasion to thank. I tried it on my young daughter, Assia, who appreciated the treatment and would run spontaneously to the vegetable garden to pick the leaves when needed. She was very endearing with her skin covered in green patches, when all the other children had red spots!

Sunburn

Arnica/Urtica dilution, for external use, and:
Arnica/Urtica gel,
are excellent local healing treatments for sunburn. At the beginning of the erythema, I recommend the liquid form, which is used to make moist compresses. Dilute 1 spoonful of *Arnica/Urtica* with 9 spoonfuls of water (use natural mineral water to avoid the presence of chlorine). Dip a gauze or piece of cloth for the compress into the liquid and apply to the affected area. Moisten the compress again when it becomes dried. This treatment reduces the inflammation, relieves the itching and restores the skin covering. In less severe cases or those that are resolving, the gel form of *Arnica/Urtica* can be used. Of course, further exposure to the sun must be prevented in order for any treatment to be able to work. Cases of sunburn are increasing greatly because of the growing habit of overexposure to sun, particularly without becoming accustomed to the sun during the hours when there are more infrared waves. The thinning of the ozone layer in the earth's atmosphere undoubtedly plays an important role in the onset of this pathology, just as it unfortunately does in the continual increase in skin cancers, which are strictly related to exposure to sun.
From an anthroposophic point of view, sunburn is a sort of accumulating indigestion of the skin's metabolism of the sun's rays. Every substance or energy that enters the body must be completely transformed and "humanised"; if this is not possible because there is too much of it or the stimulus is too strong, the body reacts forcefully, trying to expel what is foreign working inside it. Sunburn can become a chronic intolerance in subjects who do not adopt good habits with regards to exposure to sun, but also in those in whom the condition is treated by suppression, preventing the body from truly healing. Clinical experience has shown us that only a treatment that accommodates the body's own reaction, and is tailored for the individual patient with his

personal way of reacting, will lead to a definitive and true cure.
Apis mellifica D30 drops. This is an excellent preventive remedy: take 10 drops in a little water before the three meals, starting at least three weeks before *exposure to the sun, which must in any case be reasonable and gradual.*
The treatment should be continued for the whole period of exposure. *Apis* is a remedy derived from bees[88] and has a relationship with the silica process described in the chapter on allergies. It is a great regulator of the immune system and is particularly suitable for cases of allergic erythema. It is a sort of image of the process of regulation and control of hypersensitivity, which is actually the allergy, because it works by regulating our internal warmth. It is very useful in allergies and inflammation because both these processes are characterized by an imbalance in this setting.
Finally, *prevention* can be aided by a greater intake of beta-carotene, which can be achieved easily by drinking a small glass of organic or biodynamic carrot juice each day. It is sufficient to drink a small glass (for instance, a wine glass), livened up with a few drops of fresh lemon juice, starting two or three weeks before and continuing throughout the whole period of exposure to the sun. The juice obtained from freshly blended biodynamic carrots is obviously even more effective.
Other remedies that can be used in the *acute phase*, besides *Arnica/Urtica* are:
Apis D3 drops, and:
Belladonna D4 drops.
The recommended dose is 10 drops alternated every one or two hours for several days, tapering down to three or four times a day for at least one week. This anti-inflammatory treatment should not be stopped abruptly, otherwise the fire under the ashes could be rekindled.

---

[88] Marguerite Yourcenar, *The fourth name of God is "Abeille", a single word, meaning bee*, Gallimard (*Les Trente-Trois Noms de Dieu*, Nouvelle Revue Francaise, n. 401, 6-1986).

Burns and scalds

Immerse the affected part immediately in cold water to limit damage caused by the release of toxins that develop during the burn. Do not use oily substances. One really effective anthroposophic remedy, already described in the chapter on sunburn, is *Arnica/Urtica dilution* for external use.
Dilute one part of remedy in nine parts of warm water, preferably previously boiled; for example 1 teaspoon of the remedy and 9 teaspoons of water. Moisten a gauze with the solution and apply it to the burn. Leave the damp compress in place for at least five days. The compress must always be kept damp so it is useful to cover the gauze with hydrophilic cotton soaked in the same solution, moistening the cotton every now and again. This method rapidly relieves the pain and accelerates healing, avoiding hypertrophic scarring or keloid formation[89]. After the fifth day, remove the compress carefully and apply *Arnica/Urtica ointment* for a few days. *Arnica/Urtica ointment* alone is sufficient for small burns. However, in case of doubt, use the compress anyway, given its beneficial effects on pain and scarring, but apply for only a few hours.

A precious memory
I was at the beginning of my career as an anthroposophic doctor and was, with trepidation, standing in for a colleague for small routine problems. Suddenly a group of people entered the clinic. One of them was carrying a girl in his arms; a part of the child's face was completely burnt and one ear was black. In that moment I felt afraid, but the doctor on duty was me. I was helped greatly by learning that the cause of the burn was the irresponsibility of the adults who, playing with and igniting alcohol to amuse (sic!) the child, had caused a flashback. My fighting spirit returned in-

---

[89] For remarks on keloid see the chapter on trauma.

stantly and I prescribed compresses of *Arnica/Urtica urens* 24 hours a day. By the fifth day the parents of the girl were exhausted, but I would not listen to reason: I was inflexible, both to control my fear as a young doctor and because of the anger that I still feel when I remember their dangerous games with alcohol.

I examined the girl again on the tenth day and just managed to hide my astonishment. Today she is a splendid woman with no signs on her face and her father has become a good friend of mine.

This story, which is part of my medical background, has always been useful to me for two reasons. The first is my strong recommendation that dangerous games, particularly those with flammable substances, are never played in front of children. The second is my equally strong recommendation of the therapy that I have described for burns; given its efficacy it really is worthwhile overcoming laziness and carrying out this treatment, which is demanding but safe, particularly in children and youngsters.

Trauma and surgery

Contusions

A contusion is a traumatic injury caused by a blunt (not pointed) object, such that the skin is not broken. Bleeding is internal, that is, it occurs inside the tissues, and gives rise to a haematoma (bruise). Contusions are very frequent events, particularly when there are children in the house and it is, therefore, important to have a basic remedy that can be used without a prescription.

Arnica, the queen of trauma

We are in the realm of *Arnica* (wolf's bane) the queen of traumatic injuries to the body, be they physical or even psychological, such as frights or post-traumatic shock. Wolf's bane is a wonderful medicinal plant that incorporates the strong action of silica, completed by potassium, calcium salts, a bit of tannic acid and phosphoric ethereal oils. These components, which bring in the basic minerals, are used to build a sort of "scaffold for the organization of "I"", with minerals as the link, the mediator for the body within man. Wolf's bane acts on injuries from outside, because it draws the soul body from within to come to the aid of the organization of "I" in the healing and regeneration. Steiner spoke of *"a composite mixture of all the possible macrocosmic elements"*: from the yellowish-reddish-brown coloured ethereal oil (which is very concentrated in the roots although present throughout the plant[90] and is an expression of cosmic forces al-

---

[90] In anthroposophic science of the spirit, colour is the most evident sign of the action of the peripheral forces of the cosmos; of course, on a physical level this translates into the presence of different chemical substances that determine the various colours. The colour of the ethereal oil of a plant, present in the lipid part, is a physical expression of the fact that the astral forces have managed to penetrate that part of the plant. Recalling what I have already said, physical and ether forces work within the plant and astral forces act from outside; in some plants, particularly poisonous and medicinal plants, the astral penetrates into the inside of the plant. The scent of a plant is the clearest manifestation that these cosmic forces are acting.

so because of its high content of fats), to the scent of the plant (which is more intense in plants grown at higher altitudes and is another expression of the cosmic), to the sesquiterpene lactones (present above all in the flowers and endowed with anti-inflammatory and antimicrobial activities). *Arnica* also contains flavonoids and coumarins, substances which are important for the circulation.

Wolf's bane has a direct relationship with the human nervous system, which is the physical expression of the soul (astral) body[91]. This relationship helps us to understand how wolf's bane can accomplish a profound healing that is unknown to allopathic medicine (academic or conventional medicine).

The healing properties of Arnica
One type of injury that is not, unfortunately, uncommon is a *crushed finger*, a finger left in the crack of a door in a house or a car. I consider myself an expert on this matter, thanks to my daughter Assia who, as an extremely lively and agile child, left her fingers countless times in doors of houses and cars, and not only our own. If you act swiftly, you will be astonished by the results.
Arnica planta tota D6 drops: administer 10-15 drops every ten to fifteen minutes, at least for the first three hours; given the importance of the speed of action, administer the first doses directly into the mouth.
Arnica essence liquid: using a gauze or handkerchief, apply the liquid undiluted directly to the injured nail. If you act promptly you can save the nail, the pain will cease within a short time and you will not have to make a hole in the nail to allow the blood to flow out. Fortunately, children respond very swiftly to this treatment.
Subungual haematoma: in the case of a large subungual haematoma, if you were not able to act quickly enough with the remedies just mentioned, a good method for alleviating the pres-

---

[91] See the chapter 'The four constituent parts of the human being' to understand the relations between components of human nature.

sure of the blood below the nail, which causes a lot of pain, is to take a paper clip, open it and heat one end of it over a candle or a cigarette lighter, then, with great care place the heated tip on the nail over the haematoma for an instant: like a miracle you will see a large drop of blood emerging, without this causing any pain but, quite the contrary, giving immediate relief. Do not use a needle, because the tip is too small.

In summary
Arnica planta tota D6 drops: use for any type of contusion, from a simple blow to a head injury; the initial dose is 10 drops very frequently to avoid the development of a haematoma. The treatment is then continued with drops every two to three hours for three to fifteen days, depending on the severity of the injury.
Arnica essence: a teaspoon of essence in a glass of water is useful to make moist compresses over the site of the contusion. A bandage moistened with *Arnica essence,* applied for a few days, is an indispensable treatment for *head injuries* in children, but also in adults.
A doctor should always be consulted in the case of a head injury, and my advice is to go the nearest Accident and Emergency department, where there are the means for a correct diagnosis.
This recommendation does not, however, preclude the immediate assumption of *Arnica* drops by mouth or the application of the compress on returning from the hospital. Note that a head injury is not resolved simply by knowing that there are no complications, or by closing an open wound with stitches. For example, after a fall onto the chin and the appropriate investigations and stitches if needed, the patient should rest for a few days and continue the treatment with *Arnica*.
In anthroposophic medicine we do not only use the flower, as occurs in herbal medicine, but the whole plant (*planta tota*) and, depending on the specific indication, we will use only the flowers (*flos*) or the root (*radix*) because of the profound relationships between plants and humans (where the human can be considered an upturned plant: the roots corresponding to the head, the flow-

ers to the metabolic zone, the abdomen and the large muscles of the limbs, and the stem to the zone of the rhythmic respiratory and cardiac processes). You must, therefore, pay careful attention to your doctor's prescription.

For example, in the case of a *stroke* or *serious head injury*, subcutaneously injected *Arnica radix D20*, that is, a high potency of *Arnica* prescribed by a doctor, can be very effective. While waiting for the doctor you can use *Arnica radix D20 drops*, 10 drops in a little water or directly on the tongue, every twenty minutes, which provides considerable protection. Head compresses, dampened with *Arnica essence* diluted in a little water, are always useful.

For some contusions, for example *sporting injuries*, a few drops of *Arnica essence* can be poured on a piece of damp wool and applied locally, taking advantage of the harmony between wolf's bane and wool.

Arnica planta tota D3 drops: this is a remedy for small contusions, such as those caused by falls in children, particularly in the early stages of bruising. It can be substituted after one or two days by *Arnica planta tota D6* in the case of more substantial injuries.

Arnica 30% ointment: this typical remedy for contusions is indispensable for people playing sports that often involve blunt trauma, such as martial arts, rugby and football, and should always be combined with the drops, taken by mouth.

I practiced martial arts for many years and always kept remedies based on wolf's bane in my bag. Over the years I have used the drops, the essence, the ointment and also the injection, *Arnica planta tota D3 vial*, administered subcutaneously, with excellent results, as confirmed by medical colleagues who were able to witness the remedy's efficacy.

Arnica 10% ointment: this is a remedy for minor contusions and trauma, such as joint sprains, in children; for maximum efficacy it should always be used together with the same remedy given orally in the form of drops.

Contraindications: do not apply the ointment directly onto open wounds that are bleeding, because this could cause an allergic reaction.

Surgical interventions

Arnica is also very useful in the case of surgery, because it can reduce pain and complications in the post-operative period. Patients recover faster and require fewer synthetic drugs.

My prescription is *Arnica planta tota D3 drops*, 10 drops three or four times a day, starting two to four days before the operation. As soon as possible after the operation, take 10 drops every hour until the pain ceases. Continue with *Arnica planta tota D6 drops*, 10 drops three or four times a day for seven to twelve days. This basic prescription, which almost makes the use of other analgesics redundant, reduces the risk of haematomas and haemorrhages and promotes wound healing.

Staphysagria D6 drops: 10 drops three or four times a day, for seven to fifteen days. This is used from the day of the operation and helps healing of surgical wounds such as those produced by a scalpel, but also accidental cuts with knives or blades.

Onopordon/Primula comp. drops: this is a remedy that supports the work of the heart. It is used in the case of significant operations under general anaesthesia or when the patient is anxious; the dose is 10 drops three or four times a day taken together in the same water as used for the other remedies in order not to overcomplicate the administration of the remedies.

At the dentist

A particularly useful remedy for *dental extractions* is *Arnica planta tota D6 drops*, 10 drops every hour. After a few days, the dose can be decreased to three times a day, until the wound in the tooth socket heals. As for surgical operations, I advise taking the drops the evening before the intervention and immediately before sitting in the dentist's chair. An anthroposophic dentist, or a doctor familiar with anthroposophic medicine, can inject *Arnica planta tota D3 vials* into the gums or subcutaneously in the cheeks, close to the site of the tooth to be extracted.

Mouthwashes with *Calendula* are extremely helpful for avoiding complications of the wound at the site of the extracted tooth (see the following section on wounds and the chapter on toothache).

Wounds

In the realm of wounds, the sovereign is *Calendula,* which carries out its duties in a really unique way. After first washing the wound thoroughly with running water to eliminate as much dirt and as many bacteria as possible, clean the wound with sterile gauze soaked in cold, boiled water and Marseille soap, taking care never to work from the surroundings to the centre of the wound.

When the tissue has been cleaned, *Calendula essence* for external use can be applied, prepared using one teaspoonful of the essence in a quarter of a litre of water. Of course, a few drops in a tablespoon of water are sufficient for small wounds. *Calendula essence* is not an antiseptic in the strictest sense, but germs do not take hold in its presence; it is thought that it prevents microbes from multiplying, even in very infected wounds. It is used for compresses and baths, to be repeated frequently if there is a tendency to infection. If the wound is large, it is worth giving the *Arnica* by mouth, as well, to help wound healing and reduce bleeding. *Calendula essence* applied externally has a soothing effect and promotes healing.

When there is a risk that the gauze will adhere to the wound as it dries out, the gauze can simply be made wet again with *Calendula essence* every time it tends to dry, thus accelerating healing.

Calendula 10% ointment has strong soothing properties which helps healing in less severe cases, such as cuts, scratches and cracks of the skin of the hands and legs, as well as small wounds. In my experience, *Calendula essence* and *ointment* are more effective than any other type of treatment, even the most expensive.

Calendula essence should never be absent from a family's stock of remedies because it is also extremely useful in irritations of the mucosa and can be used, at the dilutions already described, for mouthwashes and gargles in the case of inflamed gums after dental extractions. The only precaution is not to use hot water. *Calendula essence* is also useful for inflammation of the genitals and for vaginal douches: the dose is 1 tablespoon of essence in a litre of warm water. Diluted *Calendula essence* is useful in children, particularly girls, who have difficulty in urinating and burning when passing urine: apply compresses dampened with diluted *Calendula*, especially before urinating, to reduce the burning (without forgetting that the cause of this problem is often too much chocolate or an excess of food rich in phosphate, including snacks, cola drinks and cured meat).

A final indication is to use *Calendula* after the extraction of foreign bodies from the skin. The ointment is sufficient if the foreign body is just a thorn.

Keloid

One common complication of wound healing is excessive deposition of scar tissue. In some particularly susceptible subjects, scars are very bulky and appear inflamed, a condition called *keloid* (hypertrophic scars). I recommend that such subjects consult an anthroposophic doctor who can be of great help. It is important not to allow too much time to pass in order for the scar to respond well to the treatments, so action must be taken in the first months after the injury or operation.

A scar is a sort of boundary, an area where the body has less control over the ether forces which stop at the periphery and this can create a sort of "black hole", a factor weakening the body; this can be called a "field of disturbance" which may require specific treatment. In order to prevent the development of keloid it is important to treat the wound appropriately and provide good general medical care before and after the surgical intervention. Finally, I would like to mention a precious remedy, *K-gel,* to apply on the affected area once or twice a day, rubbing it in until it is absorbed completely. In particularly severe cases, apply a dressing. In the case of surgical wounds, apply the *K-gel* after the stitches have been removed.

The following dietary indications are important for correct scar formation: *vitamin A,* contained in the form of *carotene* in orange-red fruit and vegetables (apricots, peaches, watermelons, carrots, sweet peppers, red cabbage, pumpkin), but also in parsley, lettuce, spinach, etc. and as *retinol* in lamb's liver and the liver of other animals; *vitamin E* or tocopherol, contained in wholemeal cereal germs, in green-leaved vegetables (lettuce, cabbage, spinach, cress, etc.) and above all in oily seeds (almonds, walnuts, hazelnuts, olives, sesame seeds, dates, etc.) and related oils. Finally an important trace element necessary for good wound healing is *magnesium,* which is present in large amounts precisely in the foods just mentioned. In the morning two or three fresh almonds added to muesli based on biodynamic wholemeal cereals and fresh orange-red fruit are a pleasant aid to wound healing.

Rheumatism and joint pain: an obstacle to movement

We certainly do not think that we are being pessimistic if we say that human beings are ever less mobile these days; think how many hours are spent in front of the television or sitting in a car and all those applications of modern technology that replace our motor activity.
There is an increasing separation between the head system and the movement system: for the most part we sit in front of a computer all day, immobile on a chair, asking demanding work from our head, while leaving the metabolic and limb system almost inactive. In the evening the situation is reversed: we leave our head inactive and perhaps set off for a run, play a sport or dance frenetically. This is understandable from a psychological point of view, but by shifting from one extreme to another we risk disrupting the correct relationship between perception and movement.
A damaged heart and circulation under pressure certainly do not gain any benefit.
According to the modern understanding of the physiology of the heart, the healthiest form of movement is walking[92], going for a stroll, where perception and movement are in particular harmony. Once it has been understood that the most appropriate movement for a human being is that penetrated by both the soul and the individual qualities, conditions which counteract the force of gravity, it should be clear that nowadays, in the technological age with its tendency to extremes, it is crucial to give movement back its central role, precisely in order to overcome the inevitable changes that occur in this sphere.

---

[92] We will talk about this in the chapter on hypertension. Movement is also part of the rehabilitation after a heart attack and walking is considered one of the relevant activities.

Part II. Illnesses and remedies

These one-sided situations give rise to the development of cramps, tenseness and stiffness, particularly in people predisposed to neurotic or depressive disorders; we have a situation in which we seem to close ourselves in a shell of tense muscles and the back often manifests the most obvious signs of this.

On the other hand, the one-sidedness induces phenomena of irritation, restlessness and automatic and uncontrolled movements, that is, senseless movements no longer penetrated by the soul or individual qualities.

The imbalanced movements of some types of sports, in which only some muscle groups are exercised, creates a specialisation, something that leads to a certain approximation to the movements of animals, which are typically one-sided and specialised, lacking the universal nature of human movement.

We can state that the disorders of movement, such as rheumatism, and those due to a lack of movement are among the most common ailments today.

Current culture has a definite intellectual inclination, it is a culture related to the sphere of the head and we, therefore, tend to processes of hardening and death.

The person who lives too much through the head steals warmth from his organs of metabolism, his feet become cold, his metabolic processes slow, his muscles cool and stiffen. Considering mythology, it is interesting that the first intellectual, Oedipus, who solved the riddle set by the Sphinx, had deformed feet.

Furthermore, modern technology leads to increasingly monotonous and uniform types of movement, the diet tends to ever increasing degeneration and mineralisation. Warmth, and with it the organization of "I" of the human, withdraws ever further from the body and this becomes cold and mechanical.

We can start by making a distinction between the disorders of movement, considering first the *inflammatory forms*, those that finish in "*itis*", for example arthritis.

These are very active inflammations that affect the joints and muscles; it is usually possible to treat them well when they are not blocked with anti-inflammatory remedies.

Aconitum/Arnica/Bryonia drops,
Colchicum/Sabina drops,
are two remedies (which we see again in the chapters on back pain and torticollis) which have a good anti-inflammatory effect; 10 drops of one of each of the two remedies are alternated every one to two hours; the treatment should not be stopped immediately when an improvement has been obtained, but continued, prolonging the interval between doses to three hours for a few days, even in the absence of symptoms.

If the pain is localised, local treatments such as compresses are useful, but traditional oils for anthroposophic massages are also valuable. For neuralgic-type pain, I mention *Aconitum comp. oil*, which is also very effective when applied along the course of the inflamed nerve. For example, in the case of *intercostal pain,* apply the oil starting from the back and continuing along the costal pathway of the nerve and muscles to the sternum or lower part of the rib cage. *Arnica comp./Formica oil* is useful for applications to inflamed joints and muscles. Your anthroposophic doctor will prescribe you the more important remedies for subcutaneous administration which are extremely effective.

Obviously, the diet should also be modified, limiting excess animal proteins and drastically reducing products of the Solanaceae or nightshade family of plants (tomatoes, aubergines, peppers, potatoes) above all in the cold, damp seasons; it is useful to follow a diet based on raw food.

One valuable remedy is *Birch syrup* to be taken in cycles lasting two months (two or three tablespoons a day diluted in water), juice or a herbal tea in autumn or spring as a treatment for sclerosis and ageing; this remedy is important for the prevention of all types of rheumatic illnesses.

The chronic degenerative disorders affecting the joints are more difficult to deal with. These disorders also affect cartilage and require prolonged treatment. They are disorders related to a predominance of the cooling forces of the upper pole. In such cases it is useful to work on the regenerative and rebuilding forces of the metabolic pole; you should contact your anthroposophic doctor who will help you by using certain combinations of sulphur, phosphorus or metals which are also appropriate for treatment of the liver.

Aconitum/Arnica/Betula drops: this is a basic remedy for rheumatic joint disorders that are beginning to become chronic. A suggested dose is 10 drops before the three meals for at least two or three months. The application of the oils described above is also useful in the case of chronic arthritis, for example osteoarthritis of the knee, in which *Cartilago/Mandragora comp. ointment* is even more effective, applied every day and covered with a wool compress. The famous ointment for rheumatism, *Sal Maris comp. ointment,* is also valuable for cases of osteoarthritis of the small joints of the hands and feet, and should be used long term.

A *clay poultice* is very useful for inflamed joints such as the hips, knees and shoulders. Use *green clay* diluted in warm water, trying to keep it fairly thick; apply a layer of about two centimetres on the joint affected, cover it, and leave the poultice in place for at least half an hour but better still for an hour. Wash away the poultice with warm water and then apply one of the above mentioned oils (*Aconitum comp. oil* or *Arnica comp./Formica oil*), or simply *Arnica oil*, which also helps to counteract the drying action of the clay.

There are also products such as *Mud Cream* which are preparations based on clay and essential oils of arnica, camphor, turpentine, etc. which are very useful for the back, shoulders and elbows.

Wool clothing plays a favourable role because of its action in supporting the warmth body. It is now becoming possible to obtain biodynamic wool[93] which gives us optimism for the future of our joints, but also for the good of the Earth. The wool comes from Australia, a country made even more into a desert by the arrival of immigrants from the western world, but where biodynamic agriculture is now developing more strongly.

---

[93] This is identified by the Demeter mark of biodynamic quality.

Osteoarthritis often has an origin in the distant past of a patient's biography; certain shocks or limitations of movement, for example during the school period, prevent the soul from manifesting itself correctly through the body, establishing the conditions for precipitation of mineral salts within the joints, a process related to the onset of the disorder. We must bear in mind that we continuously run the risk that life, that it is to say warmth, withdraws from our body, given the specific technological trends of modern civilisation; both physically and from the point of view of the soul we risk entering into dynamics of a mechanical nature. For this reason it seems increasingly important for the movements of the soul and of the body to find a precise correlation, in order to engage the activity of the "I" and warmth. As a doctor I am worried about mechanical exercises that are too one-sided, such as "body building" and certain dancing which, by following a type of muscular fetishism, can lead to a mechanisation of the movements and, consequently, also of the qualities of the soul: our health certainly cannot benefit from such movements.

Finally, I shall never tire of repeating that a diet too rich in animal proteins and Solanaceae in the cold, damp seasons is a glaring error of modern eating habits and is reflected by the high frequency of rheumatic illnesses.

I would like to present some of the main remedies used for rheumatic joint pains. They can be used alone or in alternation, although you should not use more than two remedies. Take 10 drops every two or three hours, or even every hour in very acute cases.

Bryonia D6 drops: these are useful if the patient cannot support even the slightest movement and if his pain is relieved by immobility and pressure on the tender area. This is generally the case for all pains of "rheumatic" origin; it should be noted that many similar pains appear only in some seasons or climatic and atmospheric conditions, such as when it is cold and wet.

Rhus toxicodendron D6 drops: these drops are useful if the pain decreases with movement: that is, after initial stiffness, the joint movements improve with "warming up".

Rhododendron ferrugineum D6: this is a specific remedy for rheumatic conditions that appear after exposure to damp environments or cold, wet weather.

Dulcamara D6 drops: this remedy, on the other hand, should be used in cases that the pain characteristically appears when there is a change in weather (wind, rain, storms).

Apis D3 drops: these drops are indicated when the joint is red and swollen and the skin is tender to touch, which are all signs of an acute rheumatic disorder of the joint. Take the drops several times a day until the painful swelling and inflammation disappear; this remedy should, of course, be combined with a diet with a low protein content.

Muscle cramps

Muscle cramps are involuntary, spastic, painful contractions of the muscles, particularly those of the calf, thigh, hand and foot. They do not usually last a long time and resolve spontaneously.
Only recurrent muscle cramps require individual treatment. Here we would like to give some tips on how to relieve the symptoms. Cramps may be an expression of problems with posture, particularly of the backbone, if they occur during sleep. In this case, manipulation of the spinal vertebrae can be very useful. Often cramps are the consequence of prolonged or excessive use of muscles, particularly if associated with cooling of the body, as occurs when swimming in cold water, because the build-up of lactic acid exceeds the capacity of the circulating blood to dispose of this acid. They can also be due to a loss of mineral salts as a result of profuse sweating, vomiting or diarrhoea. The first rule is to make the opposite movement to that which caused the cramp. Maximum relaxation of the muscles involved is always useful.
For example, if we have cramp in a hand, the strategy is to stretch and bend the fingers backwards by pressing on the fingertips; the same holds true for the foot. If the calf is affected, the leg should be held stretched out and the foot bent towards the knee. For cramps in the thigh, make the affected person sit on the floor and lift the leg by the heel, while using the other hand to press on the knee.
To replenish a loss of mineral salts, dissolve some sea salt in warm water and drink it in small sips. Obviously the well-known *magnesium-* and *potassium-based rehydrating solutions* are also effective and more pleasant. Rubs with *Cuprum 0.4% ointment* once a day for at least twenty to thirty days are useful. *Cuprum 0.4% / Tabacum D6 ointment* is also very effective.
I usually recommend massaging the calves in all cases, in addition to the specific site of the cramps. The calf is an area of muscle particularly strongly related to the copper process, always con-

nected to spasms and contractures as a localised expression of the astral body's excessive hold. The calf is the area most frequently affected by cramps.

Good help can come from using *Urania's copper insoles* in the shoes; these are a typical anthroposophic treatment, consisting of strips of leather impregnated with copper powder.

They should be used for a long time (at least six months), moving them from one pair of shoes to another.

Of course, keeping the legs well covered during the cold period is often a cure in itself.

One valuable indication regarding the diet is to cut back or stop drinking coffee, because excessive intake of caffeine facilitates the development of cramps.

Torticollis: a praise of slowness

Torticollis (wry-neck) is an acute state of painful muscle spasm due to atmospheric factors (cold or wind), bad posture and/or staying in the same position for a long time, sudden movements, efforts or stress. The symptoms are very intense pain in the neck, with marked limitation of movement of the joints and contracture of the trapezius muscle between the shoulders and the sternocleidomastoid muscle between the shoulder and the neck. Characteristically, the head is bent towards the side of the contracted muscle.

The best medicine for torticollis is time, time given to yourself. Here we have a disorder which expresses a gesture related to rest, as can also be understood from the position which the affected individual's head forces the person to assume. In severe cases of spasmodic torticollis the patient is forced to remain in bed lying on the affected side for about seven days, or even as long as to develop bedsores. I am talking about something that I know well: in fact I suffered from this problem in the first thrilling years of my career and it was the most painful experience of my life. I tried many treatments, but the spasm always returned until I understood the message: I learnt to go to bed an hour earlier in the period of greatest work for a doctor, that is, when there are the cases of influenza, acute illnesses and allergies in the spring. Thirty years have passed, but I still remember the violence of the spasms and I have been left with a great passion to help other people who suffer from neck pain. *Remember: torticollis and neck pain in very active people will not heal without involving the medicine called "time", the quality and quantity of the affected person's sleep.*

One useful treatment can be a combination of two archetypal remedies for rheumatic inflammation: *Aconitum/Arnica/Bryonia drops* and *Colchicum/Sabina drops*. Administer 10 drops of one or other of the remedies in a little water and alternate the two every one or two hours depending on the intensity of the pain.

It is useful to massage the neck and shoulder with *Arnica*

comp./Cuprum oil: use wide, gentle movements, drawing inspiration from the sea that massages us on a beach.
In order to enhance the action of the oil, we can apply it after having warmed the neck by massaging it with a brush with soft vegetal bristles or gently with a horsehair glove.

In the case of a suspected lesion caused by a sudden movement of the neck, for example to avoid a fall, it can be useful to wear a *neck collar* for a few hours a day. A neck collar becomes essential in cases of severe trauma caused by a car accident, for example in the classical "whiplash" trauma to the neck, when medical and physiotherapeutic care is also indispensable. There are some useful remedies to add to the preceding or to use initially alone if the symptoms are well defined. In mixed cases, two remedies can be combined, for example *Rhus toxicodendron* and *Bryonia*, which can be alternated every one or two hours if movement causes severe pain.

Rhus toxicodendron D6: 10 drops every two hours, for pain that improves with movement, after initial difficulty, and worsens with immobility.

Bryonia D6: 10 drops every two hours, for pain worsened by even the slightest movement.

Dulcamara D6: 10 drops every two hours, for torticollis caused by exposure to cold and damp.

Ruta D6: 3 granules every two hours, for torticollis following massages or manipulation of the back.

Aconitum D4: 10 drops every two or three hours, for torticollis that develops after exposure to dry cold or to wind.

The dose should be decreased gradually as the symptoms decrease or disappear. I advise against sudden suspension of the treatment, in order to avoid exacerbations of the spasm which can be difficult to treat.

An anthroposophic doctor may also prescribe very effective remedies for subcutaneous injection, indicating the injection points which promote relaxation of contracted, inflamed muscles. These are remedies based on *Arnica, Magnesium phospho-*

ricum and *Formica, Bryonia, Rhus toxicodendron*, prescribed according to the clinical picture and the patient's constitution. I warmly recommend overcoming any resistance to subcutaneous injections, which are well tolerated by practically everyone.

Exercises for the neck
As for all the systems of posture and movement, there are some very useful physical exercises for the neck, ranging from those that can be carried out autonomously to the subtleties of *eurythmy therapy*[94], which requires the presence of a therapist and offers the patient the opportunity to participate consciously in the healing process. This therapy is prescribed by an anthroposophic doctor: of course, we only want to give a simple indication, which certainly does not replace the help of a physiotherapist. Obviously, these movements are helpful for preventing inflammation of the neck and are not indicated in the acute phase. For example, some simple exercises that increase the flexibility of the neck and strengthen its muscles are:
– sit holding your back straight with your hands in your lap. Push your buttocks against the chair and your head towards the ceiling. Then bring your chin to the chest and relax completely. Return your chin slowly back to the initial position. Repeat several times, then:
– raise your chin towards the ceiling: you will feel the front part

---

[94] Eurythmy is an anthroposophic discipline in which words and even music can be expressed through motor organs or movement, thereby becoming visible words and music. It is primarily an art, represented by some stage groups in theatres across the world. It is, however, also a healthy exercise, practised in all Waldorf schools from nursery classes to upper school, and is a formidable source of health, as well as being the safest form of preventing scoliosis, dental caries and myopia. Finally, as eurythmy therapy, it is a medical discipline exercised by professionals qualified in eurythmy after five years of full-time, very demanding training and at least one year of pre-registration experience working in an anthroposophic therapy centre or hospital. It is an exceptional therapeutic weapon in the hands of the doctor who prescribes it for his patient and works with the eurythmy therapist. There are numerous indications, ranging from support for the cancer patient to back problems, from heart disorders to other serious organic diseases, and including debilitating illnesses and anxiety.

of the neck becoming taut: hold the position for a few breaths, then return the chin slowly to the initial position;
– incline your head laterally towards your right shoulder and leave the weight of your head to pull on the left side of the neck without raising your left shoulder. Slowly bring your right hand to your left ear to increase the tension, but without exaggerating: the position should not hurt. Hold the position for a few deep breaths and repeat the exercise on the other side.

Chronic neck pain

We have talked about acute neck pain such as torticollis, but there are also very frequently states in which the neck hurts and the pain disappears and reappears at short intervals without any precise reason, or can be silent for a long time and then suddenly become acute. We are speaking of cervical pain, which tends to become chronic if not treated and be present continuously interspersed with occasional acute exacerbations.

My experience teaches me that to help the neck, which so often suffers in our society, we must work to counteract fast movements and sudden accelerations. It is a good habit to try to carry out simple movements very slowly to create a peaceful dialogue with our support structures, which rest only during sleep. Sometimes we can feel that it is difficult to move the neck very slowly in a gradual manner and that we actually make lots of very small, jerky movements, a sign that we have to slow down too frantic a rhythm. It is a sign that we must use the neck to "perceive" space and work together with the sight to discover and appreciate the beauty that we still do not know, because, with our seized up muscles, we chase time that escapes us always. In this regard, I recommend reading the chapter on anxiety and insomnia and considering these issues in more depth.

Low back pain: lumbago

Backache is one of the leading causes of absence from work. The affected person faces a tortuous diagnostic and therapeutic journey; often the patient shuttles backwards and forwards between one specialist and another, from the orthopaedist to the physiotherapist, from the radiologist to the neurologist. Faced with this disorder, once again we become aware just how important a general doctor is, a doctor of the entire person who considers the overall, marvellous structure of the spinal column in the context of that whole individual's reality, of that protagonist of human life that the back "supports". Discomfort from a given part or section of the spinal column does in fact belong to the personal history of each one of us. During their profession, all doctors see many patients whose back pain is temporarily resolved by spasmolytics and mild sedatives[95].
Anthroposophic medicine considers the achievement of an upright position as a visible manifestation of the specificity of the

---

[95] I would like to mention the March 2002 issue of the "Journal of Bone and Joint Surgery" which publishes a scientific study entitled *Somatisation predicts the outcome of treatment in patients with low back pain* from the University of Mainz. Experts in spinal surgery (orthopaedists and neurosurgeons) criticised the exasperated tendency to request expensive investigations (computed tomography - CT, or magnetic nuclear resonance - MRI) and resort to "luxury" surgery (microdiscectomy, laminectomy, dynamic vertebral stabilisation, arthrodesis, prosthetic discs, etc.) for patients with low back pain, arguing that the main and most frequent cause of "back pain" is psychosomatic. Psychological stresses create muscle contractions which are at the origin of the low back pain (but also, the authors believe, cervical and middle back pain). Indeed, they even state that the solution lies in the inner search of the patient, who needs psychological or psychiatric support, not orthopaedic or surgical interventions. It seems a dream to read that the most rigorous forms of medicine are now understanding the need to treat the soul. These concepts, which anthroposophic medicine has been expressing for decades, are very gradually gaining ground, to the benefit of the patient, but also to the finances of the health care system: no country, even the richest, can afford such expensive, unnecessary investigations and operations for an existential distress that is expressed by backache.

human condition. It is precisely the upright position that distinguishes the human being as the fourth kingdom of nature: the carrier of "I", of a personal history, of a biography.

The upright position, which expresses the opportunity for the "I", for our spiritual element, to act at great depth in the body, is the source of the fundamental drive to human evolution: from the use of the thumb to lateralisation of the body (that is, being left-handed or right-handed), to the use of words to communicate and to the conquest of self-conscious thinking.

For these reasons, back pain cannot simply be dealt with as a problem of bones or joints: our posture expresses our dreams and our disappointments, even our memories are evoked by a body movement or stance, just as when we were youngsters and a certain song reminded us of that timid girl who made our heart beat so fast. We have great respect for the specialists who carefully describe the problems of a segment of the spinal column, but in order to treat the back, we need understanding, in the broadest sense of the word.

We want to give voice to such an obvious alarm bell as acute low back pain, a pain that prevents us from moving but is almost always considered as an event extraneous to the existential vicissitudes of the owner of that back. After days of mild pain, a warning that is often not listened to, one morning we wake up and find we cannot get up, or, while we try to get a box from the shelf in the office, we are struck by a searing pain in the back, like being "knifed", a pain so acute as to prevent any movement of the trunk.

Often the pain does not diminish, indeed it seems to worsen, and spreads to a buttock and the back of a leg, and no position can give any relief: even the slightest movement is enough to sharpen the stabbing pains. Strange sensations appear, likened to "electric shocks" along the leg. When examined by the doctor, there is marked tenderness in the lumbar region, and often the foot reflexes on the side of the painful leg have been lost: this indicates that the inflammation has affected the sciatic nerve and treatment is needed to resolve the acute problem.

An anthroposophic doctor, or in any case a doctor, is needed to make the diagnosis and prescribe appropriate treatment.
This is, however, an event that is part of us and that tells us that we should change our style of life before the pain transforms into an organic disorder.
Often the degeneration of an intervertebral disc, which can lead to a disc herniation, is preceded by a history of repeated back ache that was neglected or only treated in its acute phase. I, therefore, recommend that you do not underestimate back pain: trying to change your lifestyle implies giving a profound meaning to the symptoms being experienced.
Anthroposophic medicine offers numerous opportunities in this field. These range from subcutaneous injections given close to the affected joint, based on the classical remedies for rheumatic disorders and osteoarthritis, such as *Arnica, Betula, Rhus toxicodendron, Bryonia*, to remedies of animal origin, such as *Formica, Apis* and *Vespa*.
When there are alterations to an intervertebral disc, these remedies should be accompanied by preparations of disc-extracts and from the nodes of bamboo together with metals (for example: *Disci comp. cum Argento*) which gives impressive results in the recovery of intervertebral discs. Anthroposophic physiotherapy is also fundamental. Such physiotherapy includes *Hauschka's rhythmic massage*, which works with healing movements that interact with us and makes us more aware of modern day stimuli that are harmful to the spinal column, such as unhealthy vibrations (driving a car) and unnatural postures (sitting in front of a computer). Maybe we will learn to get up from a chair or out of a car for a minute to observe the dawn and splendour of nature. At risk of being repetitive, I would like to mention *eurythmy* again, the "visible word", a sort of conscious movement that is a real, deeply based preventive treatment for the whole range of postures of the human being. If the working world could and would incorporate eurythmy, there would be an incalculable benefit for health. For this reason, eurythmy is an integral part of anthroposophic activities, from schools to factories.

Going back to lumbago, the anthroposophic doctor will prescribe *eurythmy therapy*[96] together with *Disci* preparations, which often enable re-balancing of even advanced stages of the disorder.

Back pain: some practical advice
The acute form of back pain is usually the consequence of a brusque extension of the trunk, as occurs when lifting a weight from the ground or getting up from a lying position. An affected person describes a feeling of tearing or violent burning, which prevents any attempts to straighten the body. Often the person arrives at the doctor bent forwards in pain. In the chronic form the pain has been present for a long time, sometimes interspersed by acute attacks of lumbago. There are usually some positions that worsen or improve the pain, and it is useful to tell the anthroposophic doctor about these in order that he can prescribe the most appropriate remedy. One of the positions that exacerbate back pain most is sitting in a car, particularly for long journeys. The feeling of leaning to one side is classical; this is a natural defence reaction of the back muscles, which tend to protect the painful part by contracting in an attempt to hold the affected part of the spinal column still and reduce stresses on it. It is important to understand how to modify the posture of the body during work and to learn how to change position to "unload" the stresses.
Care must be taken not only when standing upright, but also when sitting, when it is important not to overload the lumbar region: chairs have been designed with back rests precisely to reduce the load on the lower back, since this load can be very considerable when sitting on the front edge of a seat.
A light diet with a low protein content, as already described for cold-related illnesses, and drinking more (drink little but often, particularly beverages at room temperature or warm ones, but never cold) are very useful for all forms of acute pain.

---

[96] Eurythmy therapy, as already stated, is carried out by a specially trained eurythmy therapist.

Low back pain: lumbago

A first therapeutic approach consists of the two remedies for acute rheumatism already described for torticollis:
Aconitum/Arnica/Bryonia drops,
Colchicum/Sabina drops.
Take 10 drops of one of the two remedies, alternated every hour, until the symptoms abate. If the symptoms improve, gradually reduce the dose frequency to every two hours and then every three hours. It is better not to stop the treatment abruptly, even if this means prolonging the dose interval to every four hours for a few days, in order to control the symptoms when you begin carrying out more complex movements of the back.
A good herbal remedy is *devil's claw*[97], 30 drops every three or four hours in a large amount of water; this remedy is even more effective if it is combined with other anti-rheumatic plants, such as willow, which contain salicylates, the active ingredient of aspirin (acetylsalicylic acid). A good preparation is *Devil's claw comp*. The recommended dose is 30 drops every three hours, or 120 drops in a litre of water to be drunk during the course of the day. This latter prescription is particularly interesting because, as we said, it is useful to drink in cases of lower back pain in order to stimulate diuresis to eliminate the metabolic waste products that accumulate in inflamed muscles. Clinical experience indi-

---

[97] *Harphagophytum procumbens*, known as "devil's claw", is a herbaceous perennial that grows in the south and west of Africa, and is particularly widespread in the savannah and the Kalahari desert. This plant has large, spherical tubers and funnel-shaped flowers of various colours ranging from red to violet. The fruit is hard and thorny. This plant is used in folk medicine for various indications, including rheumatic disorders. Some studies have shown that it has anti-inflammatory and analgesic properties, whilst others have challenged these findings. These conflicting results reflect the fact the plant has a different mechanism of action from the commonly used synthetic anti-inflammatory drugs but also that you need to use good quality products. It confirms that adequate treatment with non-conventional medicine requires greater collaboration between doctor and pharmacist, enriching the work of both. The patient is given the task of respecting the doctor's prescription and valuing the work of good pharmacists by overcoming the temptation of convenience: it is better to walk a little further and buy products from a pharmacist that has earned our trust.

cates that the great "transgressions" which are harmful to the back occur during the major festivities.

One useful symptomatic remedy in the very earliest stage of acute back pain is *Rhus toxicodendron D3 drops*, 10 drops every one or two days, followed by *Rhus toxicodendron D12 drops*, 10 drops every two hours, excellent for backaches which improve with movement after initial difficulty, and are worsened by immobility; this remedy is also useful for those forms in which the pain irradiates down the leg, such as when there is inflammation of the sciatic nerve.

Aconitum comp. oil is particularly indicated in the case of neuralgic pain, such as that described.

Arnica oil is a useful aide for long-term massages, particularly of connective tissue. Even without a physiotherapist we can use the *system of "warm patches"* to increase the effect; that is, massage the oil until it is absorbed and then apply patches of old woollen jumpers, warmed with an iron (the patches only remain warm for a few seconds, so you must have at least two at hand to alternate several times) to make the oil more effective. A good system for treating lumbago when you have absolutely no other remedy in the house is to put a folded woollen blanket on the back and then have someone "*iron" your back* with a warmed (unplugged) iron, just as when you ironing something normally. You need to find the right thickness of the blanket that lets a bit of heat pass through. This dry heat with a weight that moves along the back is very beneficial. It is a treatment that I have suggested over the telephone many times to distant patients, but it can obviously only be used if the patient has another person to help him; furthermore, it cannot be used if the back pain develops after an injury or worse, if there are wounds or sores.

Childhood illnesses

Anthroposophic medicine considers that many illnesses are not simply a problem related to the immaturity of the immune system, but that they are also an opportunity for the development of the soul and spirit of an individual. The doctor's experience as well as the patient's confirms that this point of view, which so strongly contrasts with prevailing beliefs, is extremely convincing, in particular for the typical childhood illnesses. These inflammatory illnesses have always been considered reactions to external factors (bacteria, viruses) and meet the profound need of the child to relate to the external world[98] which, in this way, becomes familiar. The other aspect to consider is that the child has intrinsic forces related to inheritance that must be overcome.

The classical childhood illnesses, such as measles and scarlet fever, are manifested by a rash that then resolves with desquamation: the child receives a "new skin".

What is expressed by the renewal of the body surface, of the body's external form, penetrates the whole being of the child, causing a major remodelling. The result of this transformation is greater individualisation of the child, which can be recognised by his developmental steps and greater autonomy. For the child,

---

[98] The current materialistic culture views the world of bacteria and viruses only as an enemy to eliminate, even though this view clashes with reality; for example, consider the importance of the intestinal bacterial flora, which is indispensable for life. During the course of evolution the various species come into reciprocal contact and tend to harmonise spontaneously with each other; an infection such as measles is a very severe or fatal illness in the first generations of the populations in which it comes into contact, before becoming ever more "innocent". In the nineteenth century, the children of native North-American populations died of measles and chicken pox, whereas now, the descendants of the few survivors of the extermination by the white newcomers, respond to measles as we do. Even the most fearsome virus has no interest that the universe (we are thinking of a human being) that hosts it disappears, because this would mean the end of the virus since it would be left unable to replicate and pass on its genetic information. Furthermore, consider how many marvellous biotechnological applications of bacteria that there are: I mention only one, yoghurt.

overcoming this experience-threshold offers the possibility of acquiring new forces of health.

The childhood illnesses, particularly the associated fever, should not be hastily suppressed by drugs; it is the task of the parents and the doctor to help overcome the illness, trying to prevent the development of complications, also by administering remedies that help the body overcome the crisis. However, there is no scientific basis to justify the suppression of a fever. Often an antipyretic suppository at best serves to lower the parents' anxiety and leads the child to look after himself less; in fact, since he feels apparently better, not only does he not rest enough, but may even stay on his feet. It is exactly this situation that puts children at risk sometimes.

The childhood infections can have favourable consequences on future health; for example, there are epidemiological studies showing that people who have had exanthematous illnesses have a lower probability of developing cancer. I shall leave considerations on the expansion of the use of vaccinations to the reader; official studies show that an underemployed immune system tends to respond excessively to stimuli and this causes a constant increase in allergies. In western countries the frequency of allergies is doubling every decade.

Measles
Almost all children would benefit from having measles; in the past children easily caught the infection when they were exposed to a source of contagion. After nine to eleven days of incubation, the catarrhal signs appear, followed, after three or four days of fever, by the rash. The measles rash appears after the rise in the fever; the face becomes so swollen that its features are changed. The conjunctiva of the eyes and the mucosae of the nose and throat are swollen and inflamed. The rash starts from behind the ears and spreads to the head and then over the whole body in patches that tend to merge together; the internal mucosae are also involved. The ill patient does not tolerate light and has conjunctivitis, a cold and catarrh in the upper airways. The diagnosis

is confirmed by small white spots that appear laterally on the mucosa of the mouth, closer to the molars. After two or three days the rash begins to fade and the swelling of the face and the mucosal inflammation decrease. The cough and the cold pass and the child tends to recover rapidly, although there is sometimes a stubborn cough and a longer lasting malaise.
The treatment of measles is bed-rest, constant and compulsory bed-rest, which greatly reduces the risk of complications.
I know it will surprise you, but our experience as anthroposophic doctors make us prescribe ten days of rigorous bed-rest and another ten days of convalescence. In this way measles translates into a stage of development, becoming a *"healer"*.
The temperature should not be lowered with antipyretics, because this impairs the eruption of the rash; nor should strong cough suppressants be used, since the cough helps the evolution of the illness. If necessary we can give *Ivy and Plantain syrup*, 1 teaspoon every two or three hours. The child should be kept warm and, if the temperature tends to increase greatly and fast, we can apply compresses soaked in dilute lemon or vinegar to the calves (see the chapter on fever).
In the more aggressive forms, to protect the sphere of the head from inflammation, we can use the classical remedies for fever, such as *Apis/Belladonna comp. globules*, from 3 to 7 globules every one, two or three hours.
Since *Apis D3* and *Belladonna D4* drops contain alcohol, they can be used to obtain a faster effect. From 3 to 5 drops of each of the two remedies are administered together in a little water. Given the frequency of the doses, it is preferable to use the alcohol-free globules in young babies. Another remedy that can be given in very acute forms is *Argentum/Quartz globules,* 3-7 globules every two or three hours, possibly alternated with *Apis* and *Belladonna*, to protect the head from the inflammation without suppressing the latter.
It is always very important to check that the child is opening his bowels. An enema can be useful to cool the child slightly and hydrate him as well as, obviously, freeing the bowels, which must be

emptied every day even if the child is eating virtually nothing. The diet consists of fruit juices and fresh fruit; an infant's milk can be "lightened" by diluting it 50% with natural mineral water. Proteins should be avoided in the acute phase of the illness and you should wait until the child's appetite has recovered before re-introducing them.

Once the fever has disappeared, anthroposophic tonics containing calcium and iron can be used. *Blackthorn syrup* is an excellent way of providing energy and stimulating the appetite, while *Buckthorn syrup* is ideal for supporting the defences and helping the mucosae. The total daily dose is 3 to 6 teaspoons given in two or three administrations in water, yoghurt or fruit juice.

Scarlet fever

This illness, which is much rarer than measles, requires constant monitoring, particularly because of the potential complications in the ears and kidneys. The illness appears without warning signs, with the patient suffering immediately from a high fever, vomiting and headache. The palate is bright red and the tonsils inflamed. A rash accompanied by itching appears first on the neck and then extends downwards to the trunk: the exanthema is very dense and makes the skin uniformly red. However, in some cases the rash is not very obvious and can be seen only in the groin and surrounding area. On the third or fourth day the classical "strawberry tongue" may appear, facilitating the diagnosis. After five to six days the rash gradually fades and a typical form of desquamation (peeling of flakes of skin) starts, definitively confirming the diagnosis. This *illness must always be supervised by a doctor*. We try to avoid antibiotic treatment, if possible, but without dogmatism. In any case, a diet consisting entirely of local fresh fruit and fruit juices is recommended for the first five to six days, until the tongue has returned to normal. Blended drinks are permitted as long as they are made only of fresh fruit, water and unrefined sugar or honey. It is important to check that the patient opens his bowels every day, a function which can be aided in small children by *Cichorium Rh D3*, 5 drops four times a day, and in older chidren by *Fragaria/Vitis*, one or two tablets to chew four or five times a day. An enema is always very useful.

Complete bed-rest must last for three weeks. My wife learnt this from experience when a pair of our friends from Rome came to stay with us in Milan for a weekend with their son Costantino. Little Costantino ended up staying with us for a whole month because the evening he arrived he developed a really high fever and had a burning throat. As an anthroposophic doctor I could not just give him antibiotics and make him travel home in such a state. Although my daughter slept in the same bunk bed, she did not catch the infection, which is just one more demonstration that bacteria alone are not enough to make us ill. I looked after the boy's treatment, but my wife had to manage two four-year olds with very different needs and notable logistic problems, certainly not resolved by the telephone calls from the parents in Rome, who felt very reassured by our treatment. Luckily Costantino was a peaceful child who liked colours, in particular yellow, which he used in his drawings on sheets of paper, but also a little bit on the sheets of the bed and the walls of the bedroom...

Chicken pox
Chicken pox is very contagious and is transmitted through the air. The rash appears even without a high fever and consists of fluid-filled vesicles all over the body, under the hair, in the mouth and on the conjunctival and genital mucosal membranes. The rash continues in various waves for four or five days, with new vesicles adding to those already healing. In some cases there are only very few vesicles and the illness is truly mild, in other cases there can be hundreds of the skin lesions which can cause very bothersome itching. The child must be helped not to scratch the vesicles because he could break them and cause permanent scarring. One way of reducing the itching is to apply small doses of mentholated talcum powder, although not in the first few days of the rash when liquid is still coming out of the vesicles. A purge in the evening of the first or second day of the illness, followed by an enema the following morning, is useful for reducing the viral

load in the intestine and for helping the body's defences. One very reliable remedy is *Rhus toxicodendron D6 drops*, 4-7 drops, three to six times a day for at least ten days. This remedy accelerates the course of the illness and facilitates the eruption of the vesicles. A light diet with little protein is always useful, particularly for reducing the itching. The child is contagious for about three weeks. Since chicken pox is very infective, if a child who is not immune comes into contact with an infected person, it is good practice to give the child *Rhus toxicondendron D6 drops*, 5 to 7 drops three times a day, until the onset of symptoms (if they occur), and continue the treatment for two weeks. This advice also applies to adults who are not immune, but in their case increasing the dose to 10 drops three times a day.

Rubella (German measles)
This is a mild illness that does not require any specific treatment, except monitoring the lymph nodes, particularly those of the neck, which are typically enlarged: this is an important sign when making the diagnosis. Complete isolation is not necessary and after ten days the child can go back to school. Immunisation is permanent. The exanthema sometimes resembles the patchy rash of measles, whereas at other times it is more similar to the numerous spots of scarlet fever. A good remedy is *Pulsatilla D6*, 4-7 drops three or four times a day for seven or eight days.
A rubella infection caught by a pregnant woman in the first few months of her pregnancy can cause malformations of the embryo. I remember that a young father arrived one morning in my surgery without an appointment. He wanted me to examine his daughter Rachele who had a slight cold and told me that he had come rather than his wife because she was pregnant. I examined Rachele and found that she had very enlarged lymph nodes in her neck. Continuing my examination I also saw some small spots. I had no doubt and having enquired and discovered that the mother had never had rubella, I left the father astonished by decreeing that the child could not go home. She was transferred directly to her grandfather and for over a month did not see her mother,

who telephoned her continuously. Her younger brother is now a healthy adult and everything went well.

Since then I always recommend that young women have serological tests well before a pregnancy to check their own immunity status and, if negative, to get a vaccination.

Mumps

This is another very contagious illness, but does not affect very young infants and rarely recurs. Together with a fever, which can sometimes be high, a pasty swelling of the parotid glands develops. This swelling starts on one side from the angle of the jaw and extends towards the ear, deforming the face. The gland is tender to touch and chewing becomes painful. Other salivary glands (submaxillary and sublingual) can also be involved sometimes. If the illness develops after puberty, there may be complications such as inflammation of the meninges (meningitis) and, in males, inflammation of the testicles (orchitis). Mumps should not be ignored; the child must stay in bed for as long as he has a fever. The mouth must be rinsed frequently with a *sage tea* flavoured with a few drops of *fresh lemon,* or with a mouthwash such as *Ratamirp A.S.*, 5-10 drops in half a glass of water. Bowel movements, I shall never tire of saying, must be kept regular. *Archangelica ointment* should be applied to the gland which should be protected by a cotton dressing. A good remedy is *Barium citricum D6 trit.*, a small pinch 3 to 5 times a day for at least one week. If the fever persists *Apis/Belladonna comp. globules* can be added, at a dose of 3-7 globules alternated every two hours with the *Barium* for as long as the fever lasts, then continuing only with the powder.

Pertussis (whooping cough)

Anthroposophic medicine has particular experience in the treatment of this illness, which in the past was very dangerous. The efficacy of natural remedies is particularly evident in the treatment of whooping cough. *In the case of a young child or a baby, it is essential to obtain individualised treatment from a doctor.*

As for chicken pox, our principle is to promote the eruption, not to suppress the paroxysmal attacks of coughing, but to try to make them emerge in a less spasmodic and thus more acceptable way. There will still be disturbed nights, this is inevitable, but between the paroxysms the child will go back to playing peacefully, a sign that he has tolerated the challenge of this illness well.

A breathing disorder should always make one think of the astral body, the organ of emotional life; for this reason it is very important to provide a peaceful environment around the child. During a fit of coughing, you should speak calmly to the child without creating anxiety, leaving him to expectorate and, if he vomits food, wait until the attack has finished and then give him the remedy with a small amount of food. Meals should follow the rhythm of the coughing attacks and should always be small. Any weight loss will be recovered after the illness, when the appetite increases spontaneously. This is a salutogenic illness, above all for the astral body and, therefore, for the emotional life of the child, who emerges inwardly strengthened from this challenging, but useful, experience. In a time like ours, in which our emotional life is subjected to stimuli that are difficult to assimilate – just think of the increasing number of parents who separate or who are absent from their child's life, ever increasing work commitments or chaotic traffic that steals hours of our life – an illness such as whooping cough, which attracts the emotional support of the parents, offering them the chance to test their capacity to stay with their children, should be accepted much more peacefully.

The most reliable remedies are *Ipecacuanha comp. drops* and *Cuprum aceticum D4 drops,* which should be given at a dose of 5-10 drops in a little water, alternated every two or three hours. *Cuprum aceticum* should preferably not be given immediately after a meal, because it tends to promote coughing and could therefore potentially cause vomiting.

A light diet is of some benefit, but the calm behaviour of parents is the greatest help.

During the acute phase, the child should not be kept outdoors for too long, because excessive movement can trigger the paroxysmal coughing and cold wind is equally detrimental. A good remedy is to apply a *beeswax poultice*. The beeswax should be warmed in a *bain marie* until it is liquid; a piece of linen is dipped into the wax and then put on the child's chest and covered with a shawl in order to keep the wax warm and liquid for as long as possible. The poultice should be left in place all night.

Some benefit can be derived from a warm bath to which 2 or 3 tablespoons of sugar-free *Blackthorn juice* are added. The child should be bathed in the evening before dinner, keeping him in the bath for a short time to tone the ether body and then dried well.

For grandparents "infected" by an irritating, persistent cough in the morning, it is useful to combine the same two remedies described above, administering the drops every two hours. In fact, this cough may be a sort of latent contagion of the elderly who generally have impaired immune defences that lower the "*immune competence*" (*acquired immunity*) and, therefore, develop a rather vague illness rather than the full-blown infection.

Tiredness: giving way to the forces of weight

Asthenia[99] is the symptom most commonly complained of by patients. It is a disorder for which the classical medical system has few solutions. Anthroposophic medicine, which has a natural tendency to deal with health rather than illness, can be really useful in the numerous cases in which the treatment of tiredness requires appropriate instructions and recommendations in order that the person's whole existence can regain vitality and energy. Nowadays there is a growing awareness that behaviour and emotional state can play fundamental roles in causing health and illness. The first important step is to accept this symptom as a message of life: we must not consider fatigue as something that has descended from heaven, but rather as something that is ours, which belongs to us, like our existence. Of course, tiredness can be an expression of acute anaemia, heart disease or a tumour and can, therefore, be a very useful warning that helps the doctor make an early diagnosis. One good piece of advice is, therefore, to consult your doctor in the case of unexplained or overly persistent fatigue or tiredness that does not respond to rest, particularly if the tiredness remains or worsens when you carry out activities different from your daily ones, such as when you are on holiday, or doing something that you enjoy. We now have a new illness called *"chronic fatigue syndrome"*[100] which is related to

---

[99] Asthenia is a term used by doctors to indicate a state of general weakness of the body; it derives from the Greek *asthéneia*, composed of the prefix *"a"* denoting "without" and *sthénos*, "force"; literally meaning "lacking strength". The non-specific symptoms include lack or loss of muscle strength, easy fatigue and inadequate reactions to stimuli.

[100] "Chronic fatigue syndrome" (CFS) is a term coined recently, in 1988, to describe a combination of various, persistent symptoms: recurrent sore throat, low grade fever, swollen lymph nodes, headache, joint and muscle pains, intestinal disturbances, emotional stress, depression and inability to concentrate. In reality, the medical literature has reported on similar conditions since 1860. From that time the constellation of symptoms has been given numerous names including chronic mononucleosis-like syndrome, chronic Epstein-Barr virus (EBV)

poor function of a person's immune system and a chronic viral disease; it is a syndrome that causes many problems for both doctors and patients.

According to anthroposophic understanding, a pathological process is considered to be a dislocation of normal (physiological) process. For example, atherosclerosis is the expression of the tendency to form bone, except this occurs within the walls of a blood vessel, so the illness is a normal process that is occurring in a different setting and in a different way.

Anthroposophic medicine includes the concept of *"neurasthenia"*, a condition that develops when the activity of the nerve-sense system in its own setting is too strong and dominates the metabolic sphere, causing a reduction in activity to the point of atrophy, a sort of stiffness that limits and reduces the legitimate function of the metabolism, as the organ of movement and activity.

Patients with this condition have an unchanged perception of their own capacity to plan activities, but their ability to "put them into action", to carry them out, is compromised. Thus, the first real treatment of tiredness is activity, a new, free activity. For example, in the weekend we manage to carry out physically demanding activity precisely because we do it outside of the repetitive and monotonous treadmill of our daily life. *The real treatment of tiredness requires work: new activities that rebalance and restore the nerve-sense system so that it works appropriately in its sphere of competence.* Often an **anthroposophic artistic activity**[101],

---

syndrome, yuppie flu, post-viral fatigue syndrome, chronic fatigue and immune dysfunction syndrome (CFIDS), Icelandic disease, Royal Free Hospital disease and many others. I quote from a classical scientific article: *"just to complicate matters, the symptoms of chronic fatigue strongly resemble those of neurasthenia, a disorder described for the first time in 1869"*. One notes that official medicine, with its mania for change, often forgets having already discovered what is nowadays hailed as new.

[101] Anthroposophic therapeutic artistic activities, such as painting, modelling and sculpture, are integral parts of anthroposophic medicine and in some countries, such as the Netherlands, Switzerland and Germany, are reimbursed by Health Care insurers.

Part II. Illnesses and remedies

for example watercolour painting or modelling, has a formidable invigorating effect, enabling our soul to breathe deeply, vitalising and harmonising the whole body starting from the body's respiration. Perhaps we should go for a good walk in the mountains to breathe clean air, but it is even better to do this to see broader panoramas than that of the building in front of the house and to hear more authentic sounds than those of city cacophony. Modern immunology has fundamental knowledge that should be valued.

We now know that emotional states such as depression and even boredom are accompanied by weakening of the immune system and a reduction in the activity of natural killer cells[102], a type of lymphocyte essential for our defences.

A hearty laugh among friends, a stirring art exhibition, a good play at the theatre and, above all, a true love story, but also, dear friends, a new creative spark in our relationship with the partner of our life, discovering that he or she is beautiful because his or her face shows all the emotions of life: when we manage to rediscover the beauty imprisoned in reality we are achieving really potent medicine and giving renewed zest to our warrior-like white blood cells (such as the natural killer cells), which were depressed and demotivated by the greyness of a life lacking true emotions.

In this sense, a spiritual journey, as indicated by Rudolf Steiner, is a marvellous help, an exercise that tones our soul and precious "I"[103]. One useful exercise is to go over the day's events in your mind each evening. You will discover that no day is the same as another, and in the apparent repetitiveness of the days you can find small sparks of life and the gratitude for the tender smile of a child or the deep gaze of a loved one will become gratitude for

---

[102] Irwin M, et al., *Reduction of immune function in life stress and depression*, "Biol. Psych." 27: 22-30, 1990.

[103] Rudolf Steiner, *How to Know Higher Worlds: A Modern Path of Initiation* (CW 10). This book is fundamental for beginning an independent process of spiritual research, a true self-treatment of the human condition.

Tiredness: giving way to the forces of weight

life and the world. I do not know of any medicine that is more invigorating than sincere gratitude. Happiness is in giving and in receiving the gifts of life[104].

Some simple advice
My first advice is to avoid anything that can lower one's own self-esteem. If I may express myself simply, I find that one of the deep, underlying causes of suffering is the inability to make reasonable plans for oneself; one good strategy is certainly to lower the demands on yourself, and then lower them again, but at that point respect them, because the frustration derived from not doing so drains our deepest forces.
I often give my patients this simple example. I would like to have clean shoes, so I make a commitment with myself to clean them: instinctively I would say, "every three days I will polish a pair of shoes". Wait a minute! I must lower my ambitions, dear friends. After a long negotiation with myself, I decide to polish a pair of shoes once a month on Saturday morning. I assure you that when the day comes, the task seems difficult, but I must do it. After one year I will have collected twelve victories and, taking into account that a pair of shoes remains clean for four to seven days, I will have had clean shoes for about one hundred and fifty days of the year.
Another good tip for recovering energy is to intensify the depth of sleep with a warm bath with *Lavender relaxing bath milk* in the evening; put two or three tablespoons of the lavender milk in the bath water and rest in the water for a few minutes. In contrast, *Rosemary invigorating bath milk* should be used in the morning because in has an invigorating effect that is inappropriate in the evening; rosemary milk is a tonic that acts on the metabolism, while lavender milk acts on the nerve-sense system.
Great benefit can also be had from oils for massages rubbed into

---

[104] This phrase is taken from a small, but delightful book by Claudio Risé, *Felicità è donarsi* (Sperling & Kupfer, Milan 2004), in which the author courageously suggests that egoism makes us ill.

Part II. Illnesses and remedies

the body after the bath; for the evening I recommend the extremely pleasant *Lavender oil* which is a real blessing for the nervous system, also because the scent of lavender relaxes and tones our nervous system starting from the sense of smell. I often use this treatment with excellent results in restless babies or babies that have undergone trauma during delivery. In contrast, my recommendation for the morning, after the bath with rosemary milk, is to rub the whole body with *Arnica oil*. In the most tired subjects, those with weakest defences and in the most delicate babies, you can use the precious *Sea buckthorn oil*.

Fruit syrups are very useful and have a good tradition of use in care and prevention, although some are true innovations, such as *Sea buckthorn syrup*. This syrup is obtained from the berries of the buckthorn plant, which is a ground-breaker in the main valleys of the southern faces of the Alps and their river beds; the berries are harvested in the most ecologically intact areas, such as Friuli in Italy and the southern Alps in France. This syrup is particularly useful in autumn, to give the forces of light, as exemplified by the high content of vitamin C in the buckthorn; we can take one or two tablespoons two or three times a day, diluted in water, yoghurt or fruit. This helps greatly to resolve some coughs that express nervousness and weakness. The dose for children is similar to that for adults, although it is sometimes necessary to dilute the syrup in a fruit juice to take away the slightly bitter taste that is so pleasant for us adults, but not always for children.

Blackthorn syrup: this is obtained from the berries of the wild plant that grows at the edges of woods and in hedges in the north-western part of the Jura. We can consider it as "*a concentrated representative of vital forces*"; blackthorn berries are a typical cure for supporting the ether body and the remedy can also be used in the form of injections and drops. I do not readily renounce using the syrup, which has an invigorating and precious effect on the metabolism and is extremely useful when the tiredness is accompanied by a lack of appetite and weight loss. It is the typical syrup for children; the doses are the same as those for the

Tiredness: giving way to the forces of weight

buckthorn syrup and it is worth taking the syrup for at least one or two months.

Red cranberry syrup: this is made up of red cranberries, redcurrants and rowan fruit and is a real tonic for the digestive system, useful particularly for cases of tiredness accompanied by difficulty in digestion and poorly formed faeces; it helps the formation of balanced bacterial flora.

I have used it with great trepidation but satisfaction in children in difficult circumstances, with a weak intestine and dry skin, and in adopted children from orphanages in third world countries. Seeing these children bloom in our world so lacking in purity makes me want to give these syrups, together with a chance to practice eurythmy, to all orphans, without forgetting that love is the greatest medicine.

Birch (Betula) syrup: birch is the tree of youth, as shown by its clear, bright leaves that move at the slightest breath of air, which never grows old. The syrup is indicated for both adults and the elderly. Obtained from the precious leaves of wild birch in the unspoiled southern Bohemia, it is a formidable remedy for processes of sclerosis and ageing.

We use birch in many of our remedies for rheumatic and degenerative joint disorders and to counteract the decline in intellectual functions. Tiredness in the elderly responds superbly to birch, which is used particularly in the spring for at least two months at the doses indicated for the other syrups. It can also be used in the autumn. I advise a certain generosity in both the dose and the duration of use of syrups. Birch syrup is particularly good and can also be used, diluted with warm water, as a pleasant drink.

Taken after meals, diluted with hot water and with the addition of a few drops of *Amara Tropfen,* it becomes a particularly pleasant and effective drink to aid digestion.

Finally in patients who suffer from weakness that worsens in the morning and the evening, we can combine the quick morning bath with rosemary milk, the birch syrup at lunch and dinner for adults, and the blackthorn syrup for children and adolescents.

Part II. Illnesses and remedies

Overwork
A remedy for the tiredness from physical overwork is:
Rosemary invigorating bath milk, three spoons,
Arnica essence, two spoons;
pour both remedies into the bath and mix well with the bathwater by walking around in the bath and then soak yourself in the bath for ten minutes.

Loss of appetite
Loss of appetite is a symptom that is particularly "dramatized" by many mothers who see their maternal role questioned if a child refuses food. On various occasions we have tried to stimulate reflection on the fact that our current lifestyle tends to overfeeding, creating the conditions for severe degenerative illnesses. The increase in obesity in children is becoming an important medical and social problem.

From a clinical point of view we can say that picky children are extremely healthy and that this is a source of further frustration to overprotective mothers and fathers who have fewer occasions to relieve their anxieties, given that their children are rarely ill. Let's leave these children space to breathe and acquire healthy eating habits, a task that is impossible when there are parents who beg them to eat "just a little bit!" at any cost. I consider it an unequivocal sign of the decline of our society that there are children, and not just a few, that eat only three of four types of food, which of course include, crisps, chocolate and ham snacks, or the like. Essentially the least healthy and least important foods. A more serious attitude towards food and the capacity to control unjustified anxiety greatly help to overcome these problems. I can ensure you that missing a few meals is certainly not dangerous for a child and will help him to change his behaviour. Food comes from the earth, it is a gift to us from nature and human beings have the duty to accept it with respect; exaggerated hoarding or wastage makes our life less useful, taking the "meaning" away from life. When a child's loss of appetite appears after an exanthematous infection or important illness such as pneumonia,

Tiredness: giving way to the forces of weight

a good remedy is a *bitter*, a few drop before meals to make the astral and the "I" deal with the body again and in this way stimulate the appetite.

Gentian D1 drops: 5-10 drops in a little water at least ten minutes before meals. Those children who really cannot take the bitter in drops can be given *Gentian comp. globules*, 5-7 globules ten minutes before meals.

The syrups described above are also useful, particularly the *Blackthorn syrup,* which stimulates the appetite.

The problem of lack of appetite in adults is related to insufficient spiritual activity of the kidney-organ and of the astral body; there are also many illnesses in which the lack of appetite (anorexia) is an important symptom, for example AIDS or malignant cancers; in these cases, individualised treatments are necessary. I would like to remind you that a good remedy for adults with a lack of appetite related to periods of excessive stress or anxiety is another bitter: *Absinthium D1/Resina Laricis D3aa drops*: 10 drops in a little water fifteen minutes before meals; this important remedy strengthens the digestion.

Amara Tropfen drops: 15-20 drops in half a cup of warm water before meals; this is a less specific remedy which helps gastric secretion.

Gentian bitter for internal use: the dose is from half a teaspoon to a teaspoon diluted in half a cup of warm water before the three meals; this is effective if there is a tendency to nausea and swelling. *These three remedies are contraindicated in pregnancy because they contain absinthe.*

The already mentioned *Gentian D1 drops* can be used in pregnancy, 10 drops ten minutes before the three meals.

Anaemia: the strength of Mars[105] to stay on the Earth

Human blood contains red blood cells, which live for a limited time and do not have a nucleus. Red blood cells are produced in the bone marrow and contain haemoglobin, a protein the central part of which is iron. In the lungs, oxygen binds to the iron in a reversible manner and is transported through the body to the periphery where the oxygen is released to play its essential role in cellular energy processes. Vice versa, carbon dioxide, CO_2, which is formed during the cellular processes, is transported in the blood to the lungs where it is exhaled. Besides carrying the respiratory gases, iron enables a sort of combustion of substances in the cell (cellular metabolism); furthermore, it is found in mitochondria, units of the organism that supply energy[106] to the whole metabolism. The existence of oxygenation and the intracellular mitochondrial energy processes, both connected to iron, enable human beings to carry out actions in the external world; without iron we would be condemned to a vegetative life like that of plants, whose molecules of chlorophyll contain magnesium rather than iron. The iron not used is transported in the blood bound to a protein called transferrin and deposited in the reticulo-endothelial system bound to two other proteins called ferritin and haemosiderin. A surplus of iron induces the formation of deposits of the metal in the tissues of the liver, heart, pancreas and hypothalamus, leading to a stiffening of the shape and decrease

---

[105] In Roman mythology Mars was the god of war and was associated with the planet Mars; iron is the metal attributed to the connection between the cosmos and the Earth. Still today in some countries "martial therapy" means the administration of iron.

[106] Mitochondria contain "working units" called cytochromes which, in turn, contain iron. These cytochromes are the site of the oxidative phosphorylation that enables substances rich in energy, such as NADH and NADPH, to transfer their energy to ATP, which then returns it in the various metabolic processes.

of the function of these organs; this causes serious disorders such as cirrhosis of the liver. We can say that an excess of iron leads to rigidity and inability to finalise movements as occurs in Parkinson's disease in which iron is deposited in the basal ganglia of the brain. In contrast, a lack of iron leads to excessive "softness" of the body, sometimes necessary in particular stages of life of the person, such as pregnancy during which there is a physiological drop in iron to enable the growth of an extraneous life and to allow easier delivery of the baby.

Summarising we can say that anaemia is a decrease in the number of red blood cells and a reduction in the amount of haemoglobin that they contain. In fact, anaemia is not a single illness, but the manifestation or effect of numerous different illnesses. The most frequent types of anaemia can be divided into three groups.

1) *Anaemia due to reduced production of red blood cells*: the most common cause is lack of iron, vitamins and trace elements, due to dietary errors or defects in intestinal absorption. The cure, as we shall see, involves the intake and assimilation of iron both through remedies and through a healthy diet.

2) *Anaemia due to loss of red blood cells*: this can be caused by visible bleeding, such as that caused by trauma, by excessively prolonged menstruation, or by substantial blood loss from a myoma in the uterus or can be caused by internal bleeding which is not directly visible, such as that caused by internal trauma or gastrointestinal bleeding related to cancer. An effective remedy to compensate for loss of blood while waiting to see a doctor is *China D12 ethanol Decoctum drops*, 10 drops in a little water three or four times a day. This remedy helps in the case of haemorrhages or large losses of fluid, accompanied by malaise, fainting, buzzing in the ears and abdominal bloating. It is a characteristic remedy after childbirth, when there has been considerable blood loss.

3) *Anaemia due to excessive destruction of red blood cells*: this has many causes and accompanies various illnesses (viral infections, malaria, toxoplasmosis); it can also be a consequence of taking certain drugs or be related to enzyme defects or abnormalities of red blood cells (Mediterranean anaemia, favism).

The treatment of anaemia depends on the underlying problem, which must be diagnosed and dealt with. A pale skin and, in particular, pale mucosa of the gums, lips and conjunctiva, together with unexplained tiredness, are the most obvious signs of anaemia; in more severe cases there may be tachycardia and heart murmurs. An evaluation of anaemia includes a general examination, because the number of red blood cells alone does not accurately represent the complexity of the symptoms. The ease with which mechanistic medicine administers high doses of iron is often a cause of gastrointestinal disorders, whereas treatment of the person also has positive effects on the psychological aspects of anaemia, such as fear and uncertainty.

The role of iron becomes clear if we consider the most classic form of anaemia: sideropenic anaemia[107]. The first symptoms are tiredness, paleness and dizziness. The lack of iron, if it persists, can cause arrhythmias (changes in the rhythm of the heart), and worsen or cause disorders of the circulation, such as altered blood flow in the brain, which can be life-threatening. A stressful life may also be the cause of severe anaemia. The real treatment does not consist simply of giving iron, but involves an evaluation of what would be worth changing in the affected person's lifestyle in order that he is not always lacking oxygen. One characteristic symptom of sideropenic anaemia is precisely that of shortness of breath when climbing stairs[108]. The lack of iron causes a shortage of red blood cells and, therefore, of haemoglobin in the blood; this causes reduced oxygenation in the peripheral tissues with a consequent onset of easy fatigue.

Spa treatment with Levico water
Anthroposophic medicine attributes great value to spa treatment with water that represents real magic for anaemia and thyroid disorders. Baths with different concentrations of Levico water are

---

[107] Sideropenic anaemia, or iron deficiency anaemia.
[108] The person typically becomes short of breath early on climbing stairs, but much less so on going down the stairs.

used and the same water is also taken in small doses by mouth (from 1 to 3 teaspoons a day diluted in water, with a few drops of fresh lemon juice added). This treatment is only possible at Levico Spa or at the "Casa di Salute Raphael" at Roncegno (Italy), where anthroposophic medicine is practised.

Levico comp. globules: 10 globules three times a day; this is a preparation that contains *Prunus spinosa* (blackthorn), St. John's wort and "strong" Levico water; taking this supports the copper process and acts by promoting the absorption of iron and making it available for the production of blood; it is a good tonic that is particularly indicated in forms of anaemia accompanied by low blood pressure.

Levico D3 drops and *vials*: these are used as anthroposophic remedies also for other indications, from dizziness related to weakness following an infection, to easy fainting, and to diarrhoea (see the specific chapter). These symptoms are often related to each other.

The nailed apple

Since Mediaeval times people who needed iron have eaten apples that have been transfixed with nails; in fact, the acids in the apple (particularly malic acid and citric acid) dissolve the iron in the nail and the apple itself becomes enriched in this precious metal. A good remedy for stimulating the assimilation of iron is to obtain six to eight big, iron nails, not galvanised so that they can rust. The nails should be sterilised for a few minutes in boiling water and then stuck into a biodynamic apple[109] which, 24 hours later, after the nails have been taken out, can be eaten.

The nails are then stuck into a new apple for the next day. Do not be put off by the fact that the apple has black spots at the entry sites of the nails, the taste is almost unchanged. This is an absolutely rational treatment because, as you know, rust is only dangerous in the case of wounds to the skin, not when it is taken by

---

[109] At the risk of being boring, I remind you that the products of biodynamic agriculture are certified by the Demeter trademark.

mouth and digested, since the stomach harmonises almost everything.

The nailed apple is a useful support for pregnant women who tend to become too anaemic. There are syrups based on nailed apples, but honestly it seems healthier to make that little daily effort of extracting the nails from one apple and putting them in another.

Massaging the spleen with copper

We can strengthen iron-based treatment with copper, which has a polar action to that of iron on haematopoiesis (the process of producing blood cells). Anthroposophic medicine recommends considering that many types of anaemia do not respond to iron unless copper is given contemporaneously. There is a certain polarity between iron and copper in human beings, as shown by the different concentrations of the two metals in males and females. In males it is the iron that is predominant (iron 112 mg/dl, copper 106 mg/dl), whereas in females, the copper prevails (iron 88 mg/dl, copper 102 mg/dl). This difference is even more marked in pregnancy during which the woman's femininity is enhanced: the concentration of copper triples, while the concentration of iron falls. Copper is connected to up-building, to anabolism, whereas iron is related to catabolic forces and hardening of the organism. We can say that the male-Mars-iron and female-Venus-copper "help each other".

Cuprum 0.4% ointment: a daily massage of the area of the spleen (on the left, below the diaphragm) with this ointment helps to complete the iron therapy and ensure its efficacy.

Chlorosis: the anaemia of adolescent girls

One particular form of anaemia is *chlorosis* or *essential anaemia of young women*, once very common in adolescents and celebrated in young women in nineteenth century literature[110]; nowadays it is less common for complex reasons related to the stimulation and acceleration of development that characterise our contempo-

---

[110] The classical symptom was a young woman swooning at the slightest emotion.

rary world. Asthenic, long-limbed adolescents still suffer. Unfortunately, it tends to reappear dramatically in the period just after adolescence in the form of eating disorders (bulimia, anorexia nervosa), which are related to complex problems certainly including unachievable physical models proposed by the fashion world. We can consider the metabolism of iron as connected to the process of incarnation that occurs under the control of the forces of "I", that is, of our spiritual reality that takes possession of our body; thus iron is the metal of incarnation and of the awakened presence in the body. The metabolism of iron cannot occur correctly without the forces of "I". In chlorosis, the "I" seems to be embodied reluctantly, giving the patient the impression of feeling a stranger on Earth. This translates into a hypochromic anaemia with a low haemoglobin index. This is not a lack of iron, but an incapacity of the body to assimilate it. The administration of high doses of iron causes a temporary regression of the disorder, but only with regards to the symptoms. The classical advice to eat a lot of red meat, not appreciated by these girls, translates into a counterproductive psychological pressure.

Anthroposophic medicine has a treatment that was created through the innovation brought by Steiner to the creation of remedies: *Urtica dioica Ferro culta D2* or *D3* or *Rh D3 drops*; this remedy is obtained from nettles grown in earth to which iron has been added[111].

---

111 These remedies are called "vegetabilised metals" and are obtained from plants grown in earth prepared with composts based on these metals. The plants grown are used as compost to fertilise the ground for a second generation of plants. In their turn these are used to fertilise a third generation from which the remedy that will be potentised and diluted is extracted. Rudolf Steiner had the insight regarding this method of cultivation which exalts the therapeutic properties of the metals and orients them according to the vegetable chosen. This is not physical absorption of the remedy, whose concentration does not increase, but a subtle way of dynamically activating a given metal in a specific plant to create a new remedy. A dialogue is created, a harmonious melody between plant, metal and human. After years of exercising my profession, I am still moved and astonished by this alliance between gardener, pharmacist and doctor that the patient acknowledges when taking a remedy.

Chlorosis responds very well to this remedy, which we believe should be prescribed by a doctor; it helps the body to support the metabolism of iron and should always be associated with a massage with copper (*Cuprum 0.4% ointment*) in the region overlying the spleen.

The *Levico comp. globules* already described are also a useful remedy. Finally, in cases of marked chlorosis *Levico D3 vials* are particularly valid: this remedy should be injected subcutaneously, preferably between the shoulders.

Diet in the anaemic person

This is not the place to discuss the age-old controversy on vegetarianism and the need to eat meat to compensate for anaemia. I, however, do not believe that it is necessary to force people to eat meat if they do not want to; a vegetarian diet that pays attention to the problem can translate into an advantage for health. Chlorosis, as we have said, responds poorly to the direct administration of iron through meat in the diet.

The iron present in vegetables is affected by many factors that can promote or hinder its absorption. Biodynamic wholemeal cereals must be well cooked and well assimilated, and if this is the case they become an excellent protection against anaemia and their high content of all the group B vitamins constitute a valuable ally. The phytates present in the husk of wholemeal cereals remove (chelate) iron unless the cereals are softened in water, well-cooked or allowed to rise well. Likewise, spinach loses its iron if frozen or cooked for many hours. Certainly a good strategy against anaemia is to eat a reasonable dose of pulses a couple of times a week, taking care to soak the pulses sufficiently, before cooking them well. Green-leaved vegetables and pulses dressed with fresh biodynamic lemon juice are indispensable for promoting adequate assimilation of iron. In fact, the vitamin C of fruit (oranges, lemons, strawberries, kiwis) and vegetables (rocket, cabbage, cauliflower, tomatoes) enhances the absorption of iron. With regards to flavours, I remind you that fresh rosemary and parsley are valuable promoters of iron absorption.

Drinking coffee, tea or wine reduces the absorption of iron, in the case of red wine because of the presence of tannins and polyphenols. An excessive intake of calcium, as a result of a diet containing too much milk or dairy products, or the use of calcium-based integrators, also limits the absorption of iron.

I would like to remind you of some foods that are very rich in iron; in decreasing order we have:

sesame, wheat germ, dry beans, lentils, chickpeas, tahini or sesame butter, muesli, oatmeal, quinoa, peas, chestnuts, apricots, figs, prunes, walnuts, hazelnuts, almonds and blueberries.

Sleep disorders and anxiety

For an anthroposophic doctor the subject of this chapter could be *inner lifestyle*[112], even if it seems obvious that every action we perform in our physical life has effects on our inner life. A classic example is sleep: how often has our sleep been disturbed by a concrete error of behaviour, such as an overabundant meal! There are two worlds involved in the life of a human being: the world of nature, represented by the person's body, and the spiritual world, represented by the person's spiritual individuality. The meeting between the natural world and the spiritual world starts from the very beginning of the person's life, to be precise with the process of fertilisation: this is the moment of the union between the *bodily process,* related to heredity, and *spiritual individuality* which comes from a life preceding birth.

Considering human embryonic life we can say that at this stage the human's soul-spirit being acts as an organizing power of the body. We are accustomed to considering the soul-spirit as of a conscious nature, that is, we consider the soul-spirit life to be our inner life. However, the astral body and the organization of "I", to which the inner life is related, are also powerful organizers of the body. The embryo is not organized, it is not moulded only by

---

[112] I understand that what I write may raise objections, but I would like to emphasise that the focus is placed on preventing inner suffering. I do not want to demonise treatments, whether based on synthetic drugs or natural remedies; the point is simply to take a first step to not needing treatments. Severe depression requires remedies, we cannot appeal to the patient's will because this is precisely what is lacking. Likewise, severe insomnia or bad panic attacks need remedies. A classic feeling that I consider counterproductive makes a patient say, almost distractedly, perhaps at the end of a long consultation: "Doctor, I *have* insomnia, can you give me something?". The duty of a doctor is to relieve suffering and so we will give a remedy, perhaps trying to adapt it to the individual patient, but I would like to try to explain that it is a mistake to think of insomnia as a "foreign body" that comes from outside and can be disposed of like a microbe. We *"are"* our insomnia, it expresses a question that comes from within us. It is a request to stay awake, to talk with ourselves. That neglected person is actually myself: it is I who is asking for help from myself, only I can truly help myself.

Sleep disorders and anxiety

the forces of heredity, but also in a formative way by the forces of spiritual individuality; if this were not to be the case, then at the end of embryonic development all neonates would be the same. The fact that, at birth, we have well-defined and characteristic individuals derives from the actions of the soul and spirit already during the embryonic process. This moulding action of the soul and spirit continues, albeit less strongly, for the whole of life. The soul-spirit of the human being continuously shapes and supports the life of our organs. Considering the importance that our inner life has on disease processes, it is essential to understand the relationship between our soul-spirit reality and our organs and bodily processes. Psychosomatic medicine is limited to noting that, in the presence of certain emotional circumstances, there are some effects on the body: the heart rate increases, the hands become cold, stomach ulcers develop, and there can be hot flushes. There are words that cover up an absolute void, such as the concept of somatisation, which expresses nothing other than the parallel onset of certain phenomena. "Taking things to an extreme, we can say that we human beings are nothing other than a somatisation. What other is the process of incarnation, through which the spirit becomes body, than a process of somatisation? Our whole body is truly a somatisation and it is obvious that a change in our inner state will also have a bodily manifestation"[113].

What interests us is to establish precisely how the soul-spirit being is related to the heart or to respiration; this cannot be done by speculation, in an abstract manner, but it can be achieved by precise investigations using the methods of spiritual science described in the fundamental books by Steiner[114].

---

[113] These are the precise words of Dr. Aldo Bargero, a pioneer of anthroposophic medicine in Italy. I am honoured to have been his pupil. I would like to convey to the reader the astonishment that my colleagues and I, then medical students, felt when hearing of criticism of what, thirty years ago seemed already a major opening compared with academic medicine which only considered quantifiable data. Continuing our study, we realised just how radically critical anthroposophic medicine was towards the materialistic view and began to appreciate the breadth of the cognitive scenarios made available to doctors who follow this type of medicine.

Part II. Illnesses and remedies

Let us return to the diagram of the four constituent parts of the human being:

"I"
ASTRAL BODY
---
rhythm

ETHER BODY
PHYSICAL BODY

The combination of the physical body and the ether body is our living body, that which remains in bed while we sleep. When we wake up, the soul-spirit elements enter us, that is the astral body and the organization of "I". Going through the various states of consciousness, for example, from waking to sleep, there is an oscillation, a continuous detachment and interpenetration of the soul-spirit and physical-etheric along the line that separates the astral and the etheric. This is where the rhythmic process originates and is manifested. This interplay between the astral and the etheric, between soul and life, gives rise to the fundamental rhythm between sleep and wakefulness. We can say that the fundamental cause of illness can always be found in the disturbance of this rhythm. Before an illness becomes an alteration of metabolic processes or a change in structure, it is always manifested in the rhythmic process; thus, the first origin of illness is always where the soul meets the living process. This separation and re-union occurs during sleep. It is during sleep that the "I" and the astral body live and work in another reality, leaving the ether body and the physical body; this also happens to a much lesser extent with every breath, when the astral body partly detaches from and then re-joins the etheric. All the body's rhythmic

---

[114] Rudolf Steiner gave these indications in a very precise manner in his four fundamental works: *Knowledge of the Higher Worlds. How is it Achieved?* (CW 10), *Theosophy* (CV 9), *Occult Science. An Outline* (CW 13) and *The Philosophy of Freedom* (CV 4).

Sleep disorders and anxiety

processes are based on the interaction between the astral and the etheric. The conditions for illness are created when the rhythmic process become unbalanced. The equilibrium of rhythmic movement can be disturbed by the soul-astral part or the physical-etheric part. For example, if I have a normal respiratory rhythm but I am suddenly frightened by something, the rhythm becomes paralysed, I lack breath, I stay in an inspiratory state, so my respiratory rhythm is disturbed. If I eat too much or smoke three cigarettes one after the other, the physical-etheric forces invade my circulatory process which is stimulated with a consequent increase in circulatory rhythm. If I check my pulse after having smoked three cigarettes, I will find that my heart rate is faster than the normal 72 beats a minute.

Considering the diagram above, we can say that with the upper part, the "I" and the astral, we put ourselves in relation with the world that surrounds us through perception. Via our senses we receive the stimuli that constitute the basis for supporting the activity of the soul-spirit within us, we receive the nourishment for our inner life: truth, beauty and morality.

In the lower part of the diagram we find the physical and the etheric, through which we are continuously in relationship with the world via the food that we eat: the substance of the world passes through our physical body and our ether body. We must, however, consider that there is also food for the soul and the spirit. We care a lot about feeding our physical-etheric body, but we generally do not worry much about nourishing our soul and our spirit, at any rate not with the same care that we dedicate to our body. In many cases of illness we can really talk about *inner starvation* or *inner malnutrition*. We must understand what the soul feeds on and, likewise, what the spirit feeds on. Briefly, we can say that the "nutrient" consists in a certain relationship with the spiritual world and with the world of truth. This relationship is the first nutrient for our soul and for our spirit, for the life of our thinking. Our thinking is health if its relationship with the world of truth is correct. I believe that the sense of relativity and virtual realities that have permeated modern life are negative factors;

relativizing truth is something that affects the inner nutrition of our thinking. We must also nourish our feeling, which is fed above all by the relationship with the world of beauty. The sphere of beauty is vast; it does not just include expressions of art such as a beautiful picture or a fine sculpture, but in reality expresses it in infinite ways.

Our volition is nourished by our relationship with a world of moral values. Just as proteins, carbohydrates and fats are food for the physical-etheric body, so are truth, beauty and morality food for our inner life. Modern day man has a profound need to deal individually with his own inner nourishment. In the past there was a sort of inner nutrition for the masses and, to a certain extent, this worked fairly well; nowadays, each one of us must find nourishment for our own souls. There are analogies with physical nutrition: there is no universal diet appropriate for everyone; each one of us must follow our own path.

The great spread of allergies and food intolerance is a very clear example of how the human organization rebels against the profound contradiction between ever more personal metabolic and nutritional needs, related to an increasingly individualised life, and the supply of ever more standardised foods, exemplified by *"photocopy foods"* such as snacks, ready-made meals and industrial drinks. Thus, even more so today, the relationship with truth, beauty and morality must be brought about individually. This is a big obstacle that we anthroposophic doctors find facing us, because many patients, influenced by the world of entertainment that feeds souls with illusions (not only of winning the national lottery, but also that there is a nourishment for the soul-spirit available in pill form), do not recognize that it impossible to assimilate *beauty, morality* or even less so *truth* passively, from the exterior, without effort, perhaps while crunching chips.

Passive inner nutrition: psychoactive drugs
We are continually being presented with replacements for will activity, from the electric bicycle to various electro-stimulators for passive exercise, which are a real misappropriation of the work of

our movement system, a delegitimisation of our functional internal hierarchies. This is on a physical level, but the road we are following on the level of the soul is even more dangerous.

Psychoactive drugs are symbolic of this passively acquired inner nutrition. People are under the illusion that they can buy something cheaply that actually has to be earned individually. As doctors, we often realise that we delude the expectations of our patients who think that the doctor can carry out work that actually each person, doctors included, must do individually. In this process of inner nutrition, one person cannot replace another, although sometimes we can give advice, information, help and support. The field of inner nutrition should be considered a sacred field, because it is the field of human freedom. A doctor should not be allowed to influence this world of freedom with drugs; the patients themselves should protect it!

A real alliance is needed between the doctor and patient in order that the latter does not develop unrealistic expectations: if the doctor is doing his job well he will avoid any forceful interference in the psychological field, particularly through the use of drugs, even if this will almost certainly disappoint the patient.

Let us now examine the elements of suprasensory nutrition.

Self-education, the real cure for the health of the mind

Speaking schematically we can say that suprasensory nutrition consists of taking in images from the world. We do, however, need to take in the right images and this is a major problem of education. Nowadays we are witnessing a mass inner intoxication due to the spread of multimedia, in particular television: there is a passive intake of virtual images, many of which are deceitful. These images do not interact creatively with our inner life and, in the long run, become clutter.

For over 30 years I have been interested in and promoted biodynamic wholemeal food, but I am only being coherent if I say that there is no sense in eating biodynamic wholemeal cereals, there is no need to be careful not to poison yourself with pesticides, if you then feed on lies, on false images: this is an even worse form of pollution, from which it is very difficult to detoxify the soul.

The other aspect of inner nutrition is the need to overcome abstract thought: the type of thought that we are accustomed to by reductionist science[115] is diametrically opposite to the needs of the soul, because it is thinking without images. This sterile, abstract thought tends to inwardly impoverish the human being.

Thinking is, therefore, on the one hand a problem of truth and on the other a problem of *passivity in thinking*, of overcoming the abstract. The logical concatenations in which the current reductionist scientific culture exists is expressed in a dialectic that hardly needs our self-conscious participation; our emotional life (affectivity) is mortified, leading to a loss of control of thinking. This control should be exercised precisely by the emotions to which thoughts are bound, enabling us to re-evoke them. When we speak about psychosomatic illnesses, once called "dystonic" disorders, when we speak about the anxiety and depression that impregnate the souls of today's human beings, we must know that one of the roots of these illnesses lies in the difficulty, or impossibility, of controlling thought.

The thinking accustomed to the abstractions of science, in which we all believe, is absolutely passive and we tend to carry it out in an increasingly automatic manner: it is not us doing the thinking, but the thoughts themselves, the logical concatenations that take place within us. We simply watch, we are spectators of the external logic that acts within us.

The other danger that we can encounter is the opposite situation, in which thinking occurs without precise concatenations, according to a game of associations in which we jump from one thought

---

[115] *Reductionism:* this is a theory according to which all biological phenomena can be interpreted on the basis of chemical-physical laws. In particular, this current, which dominates modern scientific research states that the properties of a body, even the most complex, are due to the sum of the characteristics of the single constituent parts. Try eating a piece of wholemeal bread made with the addition of husks and bread baked from ground, whole seeds and you will understand just how little reductionism can pick up of life, which is much more than the sum of its constituent parts.

to another that has absolutely no connection with the first and from this to another even more unrelated thought. For example, if I am thinking about a pink pencil, this triggers the thought of the dress of a girl I saw ten years ago who had the same hair as my cousin: in this way I have gone from a pink pencil to my cousin. This game of free associations, observed within us, is something that drags us inwards ever faster, until it is impossible to stop thinking, a situation very common in insomniacs in whom thoughts spin around in the head relentlessly and repetitively. The thoughts escape control, rolling down a slope at an ever faster speed with the result that we all know: anxiety. I do not think about what I am doing or about what exists and is working around me; I think about what I have to do tomorrow, or the day after tomorrow, or the day after that, and continuing in this way the thoughts draw me further away from myself, from my immediate state of consciousness, increasing my anxiety. The thinking loses concrete references to what we are experiencing at that moment.

Another important element is related to the sphere of *feeling*: the result of poor education of the feelings and of the emotions (affectivity) is a void, an inner emptiness. The lack of control of thinking leads us to anxiety and the lack of nutrition of feeling (emotional nutrition) leads us to emptiness; the consequence of emptiness is always fear; when a void is created in the feelings, fear can enter that void. Fear is the consequence of the emptiness that forms in the central region[116] of the soul, in the region of feelings.

Finally, if we do not achieve correct nutrition of the *will* (we have mentioned that the nourishment of the will is the moral world), if the will is not warmed by a moral world, that is, by ideals, if it is not stimulated by the reality of the ideal, the result is that it becomes paralysed or, another frightful possibility, our will sinks in-

---

116 Obviously when references are made to space with regards to the soul or mind, this should be understood in the sense of function, that is, not a precise place of the soul, but a setting for its activity.

to the region of human instincts: in this case the effect is violence, the mindless force of mania. So violence, too, is a problem of inner starvation which cannot be curbed from without; to stop this, we need to rebuild a healthy inner life, nourishing the process. Otherwise, if the condition of inner starvation continues, little by little the "I", that is the human being himself, loses control of his inner life, which becomes chaotic; in particular, the world of thinking becomes confused and uncoordinated, or paralysed, or breaks loose in some unpredictable way. The "I", the human being himself, loses control of all these processes.

The astral body can be imagined as a sort of lemniscate, a type of figure of eight, where one point of the upper part of the eight touches another point of the lower part. The astral body has a higher organization that is manifested in conscious life, in the upper part of the eight, where thinking, feeling and volition all work.

When some phenomenon manifests in the upper part, this resonates immediately with a point in the lower part of the eight. This is the part of the astral body that deals with the organization of our organs, enabling respiration, circulation and activity of the liver, etc. to be kept under control. The state of anxiety is located in the upper part of the astral body in human beings, but because of the typical polarity of the astral body, this affects the lower part of the lemniscate directed towards the body sphere, thereby also creating physical symptoms.

This is the concrete reality, which can be perceived with the methods of science of the spirit, which is nebulously called the unconscious. The unconscious, or at least an important aspect of the unconscious, is the expression of the part of the astral body directed towards the body processes. This explains how a change in rhythm due to the effect of the influence of the superior astral on the part of the astral directed to the physical-etheric processes can cause a disturbance, which is the first element of illness. Here there is a dystonic process, a lack of harmony, here we have so-called functional illness. The term functional illness now acquires a concrete significance; it means that the part of the astral

Sleep disorders and anxiety

body directed towards the physical-etheric is disturbed, that the balance between the superior and inferior astral begins to be lost, and that the rhythmic process is disturbed. The situation described creates a sense of inner impotence and in this condition, since no-one spontaneously accepts that something is their own fault, the person projects this sense of impotence onto the world, which gives rise to the feeling that the world has no meaning, that there is no point in living. This is the origin of the typical suffering of the modern day soul, that of "losing the meaning" of life, described so admirably by the great Austrian psychiatrist, Viktor Frankl[117]. He experienced the tragedy of the holocaust, in which all his dearest ones lost their lives, and on the basis of the painful experience, created logo-therapy, a therapeutic technique for modern day human beings searching desperately for the meaning of life. It seems obvious that it is easier to act on thinking, feeling and volition than influence one's own temperament or habits. The most common symptom of an alteration in the rhythm between the ether body and the astral body is insomnia. When the astral does not break its bond with the etheric harmoniously, when the soul clings to the body and does not detach, we have a state of insomnia.

The other, more complex aspect of insomnia is that, during waking life, the soul should acquire a sufficient affinity for the spiritual world in order to be attracted towards its realm during sleep. If, however, the wakeful period of life does not offer the chance to acquire interest in the spiritual world, the soul will fear this world, it will be afraid of it.

---

117 Viktor Frankl, *Man's Search for Meaning,* Beacon Press.. I must confess the great debt of gratitude I feel for Viktor Frankl (1905-1997), Viennese doctor and psychiatrist who, while interned in a Nazi concentration camp, gave a formidable example of the *exercise of positivity.* Steiner indicated this exercise as one of the five fundamental exercises in the process of self-education; in fact, active positivity, that is the limitation and control of critical feelings and critical behaviours, is extremely important because, in the end, pure criticism destroys the soul from within. Positivity is not a question of not seeing the negative side of things but of also seeing the positive one, the other side of the coin.

Part II. Illnesses and remedies

In 1924 Steiner predicted that, precisely because of this sort of fear of the spirit, in the future, and that future is our present, there would be real "epidemics" of insomnia that would involve millions of people. In confirmation of the accuracy of Steiner's warning, we know that today millions of people regularly take hypnotic anxiolytics, drugs used to promote an artificial sleep. Certainly what we do before going to sleep is of great importance with regards to insomnia: it is important to deal with things that increase our affinity for the spiritual. This is the sense of evening prayer, which tends to fill us with spirit that takes us with it into higher regions, thus releasing and tending to detach the astral body and "I" from the physical-etheric.

A therapeutic programme for anxiety and insomnia cannot consist only of pills; in fact, even if pills are sometimes useful, we must broaden the approach. As we have already said, we must strengthen the "control of our I" on our inner life, starting from the process of thinking. Thinking must be connected to reality, it should not proceed by free associations or in an automatic, abstract manner, a prisoner of logic; it must mirror the life we are conducting in a concrete way and not create "an anxiety of expectation" for what will happen tomorrow or some other time to come, generating uncertainty about the future. If we manage to live with our thoughts in the present, not in some imaginary future, but in the concrete experience of the moment, then we will have a calmer inner life, that will permeate us. Steiner describes this thinking exercise in his book *Occult Science*[118]. This means

---

[118] Rudolf Steiner, *Occult Science* (CV 13). The fifth chapter contains a description of the five qualities of the soul that need to be developed: control of thought, control of will, equanimity in the face of pleasure and displeasure, positivity in judging things and facts of the world, open-mindedness towards life's events; the development of these qualities can be promoted by carrying out five fundamental exercises that, repeated steadfastly, are a real training for the soul and a means for achieving health and a profound moral growth. A sixth exercise is also indicated for a subsequent phase, which consists of harmonising these qualities in the soul by exercising them in sets of two or three until obtaining the desired harmony.

consciously exercising thinking: in your mind you consider a very simple man-made object, such as a glass, a pencil or a pin and you describe it careful, trying to connect all the thoughts that are immediately related to the object. The important thing is that for a certain period of time your thoughts must not wander from the chosen object. You should repeat this exercise constantly for a few minutes every day. You will gain notable benefit in your capacity to sleep and your memory will also be strengthened.
The other problem is activation of thinking, and here we enter into the field of feeling, because immobility of thought can be effectively overcome by anthroposophic artistic treatment. This is not a pastime, but concrete artistic work, which gradually puts the soul into movement, freeing it from the rigid schemes of abstract thought. Through artistic activity, thinking becomes more fluid and is carried out more through images than through concepts. Artistic therapy is a demanding activity but is useful for our emotional life[119].
The other four exercises for self-education are also described in the book *Occult Science*. These, together with the exercise of thinking, constitute "the five basic exercises", which are a precondition for a healthy inner development.

The sense of life and health
Another aspect to "look after" concerns *strengthening the etheric*, because the inner balance is stable if the etheric has sufficient force. The life of the ether body within us is related to the reli-

---

[119] "Without the presence of art a human existence worthy of that name would be unthinkable. The more our age is dominated by machinery, the clearer it becomes that art is the only antidote that can oppose the threat of a completely mechanised life. Only art can give our existence a truly human dimension because it is the emanation itself of the most intimate being of a human". So wrote Dr. Margarethe Hauschka, one of Steiner's pupils, over fifty years ago. Hauschka supported the foundation of anthroposophic artistic therapies that have entered into daily use in anthroposophic medicine. The statement just cited is even more topical than ever, and it is with great wonder that we finally see all kinds of courses and workshops of numerous types of expression and creativity flourishing around us: from speech to sculpture, drawing, painting, mime, etc.

gious feeling of life. This does not mean being linked to a particular religious belief, but feeling inwardly that life has a meaning, that it has a sense, but also that life is something that we have in common with other living beings. This religious sense of life involves the feeling of the unity of life, and therefore a feeling of unitary responsibility which embraces us all, so that each one of us is also responsible for what the others do. Here we truly enter the conception of a world oriented towards the spiritual and we can finally appreciate that this conception is not only philosophical, but also involves the control of deep-seated health.

We must be aware that certain thoughts destroy life, while others build and maintain life. The tendency to judge the various conceptions of the world in a dialectic manner leads to the ephemeral, to word games, to an emptiness of the soul that permeates our inner self, preventing us from being able to grasp reality adequately. The tragedy of materialism, of reductionism, of totalitarian conceptions, is made obvious by their incapacity to face reality, confusing the gift of life with the wrapping in which it is contained; we are in a sick mysticism which is centred on the worship of things, the body, money, external beauty, the size of the exhaust pipe of a car. A mystic tendency that separates us so completely from reality that even a wrinkle or a rival with a more powerful car can make us lose faith.

The truth of a conception of the world can be checked by examining the effect that it has on the inner state of the person who expresses it. Goethe, a sublime poet and great scientist, wrote: "Only what is fruitful is true". The effective criterion of truth does not lie in the correctness of the intellectual demonstration, but in the internal fecundity of an idea; we need to learn to distinguish fruitful ideas, that is, those conceptions of the world that create inner health, from the sterile ideas, from those conceptions of the world that are sources of inner illness.

Aldo Bargero, an anthroposophic doctor, always gave us a word of consolation, saying that we do not need to do great things: the importance, he repeated, is to do little things, but to do them every day. Perfection does not matter, perfection is not of this world and does not belong to human beings as they are nowadays: what is fundamental is the personal effort that we make in our journey. "It does not matter if you fall, the important thing is always to get up again". This is the challenge: "To always find the strength to continue your journey despite everything".

We will not become saints, we will not become perfect individuals, and perhaps we will not even become completely healthy (otherwise doctors would be no longer necessary), but we can make some small steps forward. The most certain way to achieve nothing, to doom yourself to failure, is to set yourself big projects, great things, major works that are outside your concrete possibilities. We need to evaluate our potential, being severe in our self-appraisal, exercising firm control on our tendency to ask too much of ourselves and restricting the field further: what counts is that every day we make a small step that takes us further forward. What is really important is this effort to be active inwardly, because from a therapeutic point of view, if we want to encapsulate everything in a single concept, it is this wish to be inwardly active that counts. We can fool ourselves and remain like hungry sparrows with our beaks open waiting for food, just as we can wait for spiritual nourishment to reach us on its own, but this does not happen, this is the greatest illusion.

"We must not be sad about this, but rather we should be proud, because it is the price of our freedom" – my teacher used to say – "and this freedom is the most precious thing that we should not delegate to anyone, not even to a doctor".

Hypertension: the silent killer[120]

Balance throughout life

The development of blood pressure in human beings can be interpreted as an expression of the activity of the astral body. In order to express our inner life we need the mediation of the blood circulation that controls the fluid element, the substrate of the ether body. For example, we use the fluid body to transport substances necessary to produce neurotransmitters and make them available to the nerve organisation; these substances then concretely produce the activity of the nervous system. The heart and brain are organs of knowledge and anchoring of our inner self.

Nowadays it is finally said that the heart supports the so-called "intelligence of the heart"[121], which enables immediate and instinctive understanding of things. The brain, on the other hand, supports the intellect and enables reasoned knowledge. The brain receives information from the external world through the sensory organs and can process it and transmit it to the rest of the body. We have an *instantaneous* emotional understanding through the heart and a reflection *over time*, "visible" in the connecting activity of the nervous system and its neurotransmitters. These two components unite in metabolic activity: the fusion of the two forms of understanding, the immediate and the reflected, which complement each other and constitute the richness of human thought, become operative in the metabolism.

---

[120] One consideration on hypertension stems from the insight that this illness, which is devastating from a social point of view (it underlies most heart diseases, strokes and often even kidney disorders), can be controlled by changes in lifestyle. For this reason, this chapter is closely related to the chapters on tiredness, anxiety and sleep disorders, which complement each other; the underlying postulate is that true medicine puts the human being at the centre and not the prescription of drugs.

[121] It has now become commonplace to speak about "emotional intelligence"; see the famous book by Goleman which introduced the importance of our emotional life for our self-realisation, but also for our health, into both the scientific world and general culture.

Hypertension: the silent killer

The metabolism is implemented in muscles which enable action; the situation of the heart is, therefore, a special one, since this is anatomically a muscle but has its freedom and autonomy, not being directly governed by conscious nervous activity.

Modern physiology teaches us that any time a child cries, his blood pressure doubles. Until now this was simply considered a reaction to stress. But a great cardiologist and scientist, Dean Ornish[122], understood that this is not a response, but a *form of communication*.

Ornish wrote: "Adults do the same but they cry inwardly. When a person is listened to and knows that his appeal has had a response, his blood pressure decreases. I understood that the approach taken so far to studying the body was limited, that there was another body 'able to dialogue' which we had completely ignored, convinced that the faculty of language was distinct from it".

In physiological conditions, blood pressure rises when we talk and decreases when we listen, at least if we *really* listen; if, however, we think about what to reply, the blood pressure remains unchanged.

For this reason I always invite my patients to come to my surgery to measure their blood pressure: I ask them to lie down and say something of relevance to them while I put on the arm cuff of the sphygmomanometer, but I have learnt not to ask questions and for this reason the blood pressure that I find is often much lower than that found when my patients measure their own blood pressure or have it measured in a pharmacy.

---

[122] Dean Ornish, *Love and Survival*, William Morrow Paperbacks, 1999. I mention this precious book by a great cardiologist and researcher who became a pioneer of integrated medicine and made a firm connection between severe illness and lifestyle. A change in our life and the nature of our interpersonal relationships can lead to the regression of severe illnesses such as coronary artery disorders and myocardial infarction, without requiring pharmacological or surgical treatment. Overvaluing physical and mechanistic aspects of illness prevents really radical treatment and, as Ornish teaches, ends up by preventing a truly thorough study of these physical aspects of human physiology and pathology.

Our blood pressure increases because of an inner state of "alert": we are afraid of not being listened to or perhaps of being rejected or mocked. Deaf people, when they communicate with their sign language, react in the same way, that is, their blood pressure decreases. This means, as we have already tried to explain, that the phenomenon involves the whole human being and is not limited to speech. Vascular alterations are a form of communication like that delightful blushing of the face of a young girl when her glance meets that of a certain boy.

We blush within, that is blood pressure rises because of interest in someone else, in the world or because of fear of not being accepted.

Albeit indirectly, vascular alterations are therefore the language of the heart. They are indirect, physical expressions of the intelligence of the heart.

The writer Saint-Exupéry clearly states this in a passage from his precious book *The Little Prince*, when the tamed fox confides his secret to the little prince: "*It is only with the heart that one can see rightly. What is essential is invisible to the eye*". There is sight that is not through the nerve or eye but that enables a deeper perception of the other; we can define this as an invisible, but real human organ of perception.

The less a person is able to pick up variations in vascular activity, the greater these variations are; we can say that true communication is a vital question and we find it very difficult to engage in an honest dialogue because we fear being rejected. How many times have I understood that I have asked something that touched the depths of a patient just a second before measuring his blood pressure, then finding a marked rise in his pressure, a bodily sign of his terror of not being listened to.

Unlike a child, our cry is not "heard", no water comes out of our tear ducts, we are induced to hide our suffering, our vulnerability, or immense solitude and we hide the treasure that we carry within us, we hide our beauty.

Some women become creative in menopause, just think of some of the great authors who have written their masterpieces precisely in this stage of their life, and become beautiful without recourse to creams or cosmetic surgery. Other women, however, are driven to solitude in this period: their children have grown up and their husbands, devoured by an adolescent narcissism which will ruin them, start looking at young women. These lonely women find that they suffer from hypertensive crises which respond poorly to even the most intensive pharmacological treatment, because the real cure is to be able to communicate and to be listened to, like the artists.

When we prevent ourselves from feeling pain, we decrease our capacity to feel pleasure; it is a sort of moral anaesthesia that also prevents us from feeling the pain of others.

It is for this reason, I dare say, that *"we lose our beauty"*.

Our beauty is interwoven with emotions; for this reason a vascular and oestrogenic woman such as Marilyn Monroe expressed a femininity that millions of women have recognized and millions of men have dreamed of and desired. We will find no cream or scalpel that will quench the thirst of our bloodstream, but we need to open the door to emotions and dreams.

Reflections on blood pressure
The deviations from normal, physiological blood pressure are hypertension and hypotension.
Hypertension is considered the more widespread illness. In its initial stages it does not usually cause symptoms, unlike hypotension which makes us feel unwell, which is why hypertension is referred to as the *"silent killer"*.
The disorder is often discovered only when damage to an organ has become obvious. As we have said, this silence of the condition speaks of its nature and urges us to work hard to make the diagnosis early.
Chronically high blood pressure produces damage to the kidneys: a quarter of the patients who require dialysis do so because their kidneys have been damaged precisely by hypertension. Chronic hypertension causes dilation of the heart's chambers, which can lead to heart failure but also to a myocardial infarction; further-

more, it causes damage to the circulation, promoting and accelerating atherosclerosis with consequent vascular damage and the risk of bleeding in the brain, eye and retina.

In elderly people, chronic hypertension can be a cause of deterioration in mental functions, because it causes numerous tiny strokes.

We speak of *primary hypertension*, also called *essential hypertension*, when no apparent cause is detected; essential hypertension accounts for about 95% of all cases of hypertension.

However, about 5% of hypertensive subjects have *secondary hypertension*, which is caused by a primary disorder in the kidneys or adrenal glands, such as chronic pyelonephritis and reno-vascular stenosis, or by endocrine disorders such as phaeochromocytoma and primary aldosteronism. In these cases the diagnosis and specialist treatment are important. We will not deal here with this rarer and less easily influenced form of hypertension.

Lifestyle and dietary rules for the treatment of hypertension and hypotension
Risk factors

Various risk factors for primary hypertension have been known for some time, although the cause of pathologically and permanently raised blood pressure is not yet understood.

Stage 1 hypertension is currently defined as a blood pressure over 140/90 mmHg recorded by at least three different measurements (although some researchers say at least five measurements).

Three main risk factors have been recognized
1) One important risk factor is *too much salt (sodium chloride)*. Through its relationship with water, salt give the nerves, the physical support for our astral activity, a point of attachment and excessive control of the arterial vascular system. Reducing the intake of salt is the simplest dietary measure that we can adopt to treat hypertension; it is useful in general even when, as occurs in half of hypertensive people, reducing salt intake is not associated with a drop in blood pressure since it has a positive effect on the

relations between sodium and fluids in the body. It is essential to reduce salt in the elderly and in diabetics, who are also the patients in whom this dietary measure does actually induce a decrease in blood pressure. Personally I believe that a real reduction in the intake of salt, and not just a simple replacement by dietary products is useful, because in this way we create a new relationship between the taste and perception of food. I always advise a careful use of flavours and spices, not only because these give taste to food, but also because they promote the digestive process, that is, they perform a re-education, a reactivation of nerve activity in the environment of the metabolism. Certainly the present day diet based on refined food and with little intrinsic taste, made like that by industrial processing and modern cooking, damages the dialogue between the human being and nature, which is the real reason for nutrition.

2) *Smoking* is another major risk factor for all heart disorders. The nicotine in cigarettes is a stimulant and a vascular toxin and causes an immediate increase in blood pressure every time that one smokes. Treatments and antihypertensive measures are not effective at lowering the risk of heart disease in smokers, whereas they are in non-smokers. I remind you that cigarette smoking is the risk factor most frequently associated with sudden death from a heart attack. Smokers who have an infarct are much more likely to die earlier and faster compared to non-smokers. There is also proof that passive smoking (chronic exposure to the tobacco smoke of other people) can increase the risk of heart diseases. *My advice can be no other than to stop smoking as soon as possible.*

3) *Obesity* is very closely related to a rise in blood pressure. In fact, in obesity part of the metabolic forces slow down and are put to rest; in particular, muscle activity, the possibility of the human to act and to be free, is limited and muscle mass is replaced by fatty tissue. A loss of weight of even only 4-5 kg can induce a decrease in blood pressure; furthermore, loss of weight leads to greater efficacy of lifestyle and drug interventions.

It is very important to understand these three main risk factors, particularly as there are now drugs that can lead to a "decrease in responsibility" because they tend to reduce the immediate need to modify lifestyle in order to limit the effect of the factors. For example, *diuretics* lead to the elimination of excess sodium and fluids from the body and in the long term reduce the resistance of blood vessels, thereby decreasing the work load of the heart. However, by temporarily reducing the need to limit salt intake, these drugs relieve us of the need for self-education, of working on our habits and we will, therefore, be forced to take them for our whole life.

Beta-blockers, by slowing the heart rate, exempt us from controlling, listening to and directing our emotions, but promote a certain loss of stimuli; in fact they can have the side effects of altered mood, sexual dysfunction, dizziness, somnolence or insomnia.

An interesting fact is that treatments based on *diuretics, beta-blockers, ACE-inhibitors* and *calcium antagonists* are practically all contraindicated in pregnancy, when it becomes essential to focus on reducing risk factors rather than taking drugs.

Lifestyle changes

Limit alcohol intake. Drinking alcohol can increase blood pressure, interfere with treatments and increase the risk of strokes.

Although some studies suggest that a modest amount of alcohol (ethyl alcohol or ethanol) may contribute to lowering the risk of heart disorders, cardiologists usually discourage drinking alcohol because of the dangers related to excessive consumption, such as hypertension, obesity, strokes, liver disorders and cancer, not to mention the risk of accidents.

The American Society of Oncologists advises against drinking alcohol, but recognises that modest consumption – two units a day (a unit means one glass of wine or half a pint of beer) for males and one for females – is acceptable. The Society also states that women at high risk of breast cancer should abstain completely from drinking alcohol. The problem is that it is not always easy to follow this advice.

Caffeine can also raise blood pressure considerably, but the body is able to re-equilibrate the pressure and we can, therefore, toler-

ate a moderate amount of this substance. However, the intake of large amounts of caffeine in a short time is contraindicated.
For example, it is an error for a person inclined to hypertension to drink four or five cups of coffee at breakfast. Some research seems to indicate a certain positive effect from drinking black or green tea, particularly because the flavonoids that tea contains have an anti-oxidant action which could, for example, inhibit the oxidation of LDL cholesterol, reduce the coagulation of blood and limit the damage caused by altered blood flow to the heart.
Also take into account that the person who drinks tea usually has healthier habits; for example, the classic tea-drinker uses little or no sugar to sweeten his drink.
An *increase in physical activity* helps both to prevent and to treat hypertension, promotes weight loss and reduces the risk of heart disease. The ideal is moderate physical exercise repeated almost every day, such as brisk walking for 30-45 minutes.
Enjoyable physical activity, such as walking, ballroom dancing, taking care of a small vegetable garden, or swimming, can be continued over time and does not cause imbalances in the body. We now know that it is not the time or the intensity, and not even the frequency, within reasonable limits, that counts; what is important is *long term regularity*. You can start, as mentioned, with sessions of thirty minutes at regular intervals, at least three times a week, then increase both the number of days and the duration of the activity until reaching the ideal of about *one hour a day*. It is important to start slowly and increase gradually as the heart strengthens.
It is not competitive athletes who have a strong heart, but *men who move with conscious will*.
I do not believe that there is a healthier physical activity for the heart than looking after a vegetable garden.
My belief is confirmed regularly in a country village in which I often spend the weekends: there are active, lucid over eighty year olds, each with their own little vegetable patch from which they obtain vegetables and salad for their own food, they are autonomous and it is wonderful to see them on a bicycle at ninety

years old; there are no carers and the rare hypertensive individuals have been taking very low doses of the same treatment for years.

I have found that sometimes great benefit can be obtained from reducing the dose of remedies and limiting salt and alcohol intake.

I remind you that, starting from daily life, we can take simple actions that help to protect the heart:
– park some distance away from the place where we must go and walk the rest of the distance;
– walk up or down stairs instead of taking the lift;
– work in the garden or courtyard; I fondly remember my father growing herbs in the flower beds of the apartment block, a small task that made him well-liked and popular among the neighbours.

A healthy diet
Improving the diet can induce a real decrease in the blood pressure if this is not too high; if, however, the hypertension is marked, drugs will also be needed.

There are no particular contraindications because if the pressure decreases too much the person develops hypotension, but this causes problems particularly in the first half of life, whereas over forty-year olds live very well even with very low blood pressures.

A healthy diet is not only useful for preventing hypertension but is also a major help to the health of the heart.

An adequate diet must give preference to biodynamic or organic wholemeal cereals, from six to eleven portions a day, which are also at the base of the new food pyramid[123].

At the base of the pyramid, close to the cereals, there are also the

---

[123] The famous food pyramid was published in America in 1992 by the United States Department of Agriculture (USDA); one of its purposes was to encourage the replacement of diets rich in fats with balanced diets containing more complex carbohydrates (starches and fibre). The pyramid was recently revised and the use of wholemeal cereals was recommended, as now indicated by numerous studies.

high quality fats, such as cold-pressed organic or biodynamic extra virgin olive oil used in reasonable doses.

Fruit, from two to four portions, and vegetables, from three to five portions, are on the second level of the pyramid. The third level is represented by dairy products, two portions, animal proteins, from two to three portions, always limited in favour of pulses, walnuts and almonds, which contain unsaturated fats that are useful for the blood circulation and for the nervous system. Sugar and saturated fats (that is, solid fats of animal origin) must be strictly limited and used only very sparingly.

The new pyramid is based on two concepts that have emerged clearly in recent years; not all fats have the same nutritional value and the classical difference between simple and complex carbohydrates, for example, between sugar and flour, is not sufficient and that a distinction also needs to be made between rapidly assimilated flour and slowly assimilated flour such as wholemeal flour.

As far as concerns fats, the new pyramid indicates that a distinction should be made between saturated fats, such as butter and animal fats, which need to be restricted, and fats of vegetable origin, such as olive oil, corn, canola, and sunflower, which should be eaten daily. The use of margarine and hydrogenated fats is strongly discouraged. This differentiated approach derives from an enormous body of information which includes correlations between specific aspects of the diet and risk of cardiovascular events.

In a famous study carried out in a large population of nurses monitored for a long period, it was seen that increasing the consumption of mono-unsaturated fatty acids and, particularly polyunsaturated ones, the risk of cardiovascular events decreased continuously, being as much as 30-35% lower than that in another group in the study who ate smaller amounts of these fatty acids.

In contrast, women who ate large amounts of trans fatty acids (for example, margarine and the hydrogenated fats present in industrial products such as chocolate, puddings, biscuits and snacks) had a marked increase in cardiovascular events compared to women who ate less of these fats.

Thus, the consumption of fats of animal origin and hydrogenated vegetable fats should be reduced, while the use of vegetable oils is supported. Personally I advise certified biodynamic, cold-pressed extra virgin olive oil[124]; when this is not present, it can be replaced by certified organic oil. We have already said that wholemeal cereals, rich in fibre, are at the base of the pyramid; these should be eaten daily, whereas foods based on refined cereals such as white bread and pasta should be considered much less healthy.

The basis of the differentiation between these two categories of food lies in their different propensity to release glucose into the blood once eaten, in other words in their different glycaemic index.

Many observations, including the previously mentioned study on nurses, suggest that the preferential consumption of foodstuffs with a low glycaemic index is associated with a better cardiovascular prognosis. In fact, the foods with a low glycaemic index, that is foods that release sugar into the blood more slowly, tend to be associated with higher values of *HDL cholesterol*, popularly known as *"good cholesterol"* for its property of protecting against atherosclerosis, low levels of *triglycerides* and a reduction in *inflammation markers*, all factors that protect the heart and blood circulation.

The last two indications that I want to share are the importance of carrying out *adequate physical activity* each day and of practising moderation in the *consumption of alcohol*.

I wanted to show that the most avant-garde part of official medicine and anthroposophic medicine have finally reached a com-

---

[124] For certified products from biodynamic agriculture I mean products that carry the Demeter trademark, whereas for organic I mean a product that has an organic label recognized by one of the agencies (for example Soil Association in the UK) authorised to certify the products. I remark that biodynamic and organic products are the only products for which the whole production process is guaranteed.

mon outlook on the prevention of hypertension and vascular disorders. I feel I can say that general practitioners and the public should follow this pathway that anthroposophic spiritual science had already indicated more than eighty years ago with its creation of healthy agriculture and salutogenic disciplines of movement such as eurythmy.

The suggestions concerning fats are easy to integrate into a Mediterranean style diet, which has always favoured the consumption of olive oil over butter and uses margarine very sparingly. As far as concerns carbohydrates, this should be evaluated more carefully. It should not be forgotten that for instance most forms of pasta, prepared with durum wheat flour and cooked *al dente*, are considered by most authors to have a low glycaemic index, which would place them among the foods to favour and not among those to limit. Therefore, go ahead and eat a good plate of spaghetti, but use organic or biodynamic pasta and in other dishes make sure you eat biodynamic wholemeal cereals.

Changing your fate

The already mentioned Ornish caused a sensation in 1993 when he stated in the prestigious medical journal "The Lancet" that adopting a serious programme of changes in diet and lifestyle can really cause the regression of heart disease. In order to demonstrate this, he made twenty people with heart disorders follow a programme that involved:
– a vegetarian diet containing minimal amounts of saturated fats;
– daily stress management techniques, such as stretching, meditation and relaxation exercises;
– support groups and psychological sessions to lower stress;
– a programme to help smokers stop smoking.

The control group was formed of twenty patients with heart disorders who received traditional treatment and adopted a conventional diet such as the classical diet suggested by the American Heart Association with a maximum of 30% of fats; these patients were not obliged to change their lifestyle but were free to do so if they wanted to.

The results in the patients undergoing the intensive dietary regime and the relaxation techniques were impressive already after one year: the values of LDL cholesterol decreased by 37.2%, there was a reduction in the episodes of angina and a decrease in obstruction of blood vessels. However, the results at five years were really astonishing; the twenty patients underwent coronarography to examine the state of their blood vessels and it was found that obstruction of the vessels had actually improved, since it was 7.9% less. In the same period the control group of patients who had received the traditional treatment had decreased from twenty to fifteen people and the obstruction of the vessels had worsened, with a 27.7% increase. Furthermore, compared to the group of patients who had followed Dr. Ornish's programme, the control group had double the number of heart problems such as infarction, need for angioplasty or bypass operations, in addition to the fact that a quarter of the patients in the group had died.

In conclusion, over the course of five years, the group that followed a rigorous lifestyle programme showed a continuous regression of heart disease, whereas the patients who received traditional care gradually worsened.

Improving lifestyle is a true treatment for the heart and hypertension; furthermore, such a strategy would considerably decrease costs for healthcare systems, a fact that should not be overlooked.

In countries such as Holland, anthroposophic medicine, which is included in the public health care system, has enabled considerable savings. This was demonstrated in a study carried out years ago in the University of Utrecht which convinced some Dutch health insurance systems to offer anthroposophic medicine, including artistic therapies, eurythmy and anthroposophic physiotherapy, among its services. This was not an act of generosity, but a justified desire to save money, as well as a clear, beneficial propensity to *cultural and scientific pluralism* typical of the Dutch society.

Appendix

The household medicine store

I have tried to show how anthroposophic medicine requires a profound commitment from a well-trained doctor, in collaboration with an actively involved patient.

The ambition of an anthroposophic doctor is to prescribe very individualised treatments specific for the physical and spiritual constitution of a given patient, particularly in the case of the most deeply acting remedies such as potentised metals and the high potencies of the major remedies. I have sometimes made brief reference to these complex aspects of treatment in this book.

I would now like to give a short list of the most common remedies to keep in the home for minor illnesses and the most frequent symptoms; they are almost all remedies that can be bought over the counter and advised by a competent pharmacist.

This list of remedies is offered because of the objective difficulties in obtaining some of the remedies during the weekend, when pharmacies selling them are often closed. I have found it useful to have a store of remedies to take on holiday, but also to keep in the home in the case of emergencies.

Preparations to take by mouth

Aconitum/Bryonia dilution
This is a remedy to use for major colds, particularly if the symptoms suggest that the illness may be evolving into bronchitis; it is useful to keep a stock at home and administer it as indicated by the doctor.

Amara Tropfen dilution
Gentiana lutea liquid for internal use
Both of these remedies are useful in the case of nausea or loss of appetite. The dose is 15 drops in a little water every two or three hours for nausea and fifteen minutes before meals in the case of loss of appetite.

Apis/Belladonna globules
Apis D3 dilution
Belladonna D4 dilution
This is the main anti-inflammatory remedy of anthroposophic medicine. Together with Arnica preparations, it should always be present in the medicine cabinet. It is useful to have both in globule form, particularly for small children, and in the form of drops for older children and adults. It is the basic remedy for tonsillitis, but is useful, combined with other remedies, for any type of inflammation or infection, particularly if associated with redness and

fever. The drops are taken together as one dose (see the chapter on sore throat).

Arnica planta tota D3 or *D6 dilution*
To use for every type of trauma, whether physical or emotional (see the chapter on trauma).

Belladonna D30 dilution
This remedy should always be kept in the home and used in the case of high fevers, particularly those related to throat problems (see the chapter on fever).

Belladonna/Chamomile globules
A basic remedy for all types of abdominal cramps, from intestinal colic to dysmenorrhoea and to the windy colic of neonates. It is also useful for teething pain in babies.

Berberis/Apis comp. globules
A basic remedy for inflammation of the urinary tract, but also inflammation of the oral cavity, such as stomatitis. If there is also fever, it is useful to alternate this remedy with *Apis/Belladonna globules* or *Apis D3* and *Belladonna D4* in drops, these last ones taken together.

Ferrum phosphoricum comp. globules
To keep in the home always. This is useful for flu-like illnesses, especially in babies. It can also be taken to prevent the consequences of catching cold. In adults it is often substituted by:

Bryonia/Eucalyptus comp. dilution
Typical remedy for flu-like illnesses in adults.

Gelsemium comp. globules
This is useful for flu-like illnesses with symptoms in the head or bronchi and with a progressively increasing temperature.

Mercurius vivus naturalis D6 tablets
A remedy to use in alternation with *Apis/Belladonna* in the case of febrile sore throat and inflamed mucous membranes.

Onopordon/Primula comp. dilution
An indispensable remedy to keep in the home and take with you on journeys; it supports the heart and is useful for high fevers, but also for overcoming the disturbances due to the "change of air" when travelling. Administer this remedy, possibly associated with *Arnica*, directly onto the tongue for a faster onset of action in the case of shock of any type or fainting.

Phosphorus D5 dilution
Tartarus stibiatus D5 dilution
The two remedies taken together and alternated with *Aconitum/Bryonia* form the basic treatment for bronchitis (see the specific chapter).

Pyrit/Zinnober tablets
Useful for pharyngitis, tonsillitis and laryngitis. It may be alternated with *Apis/Belladonna* if there is a fever or marked redness. Dissolve a tablet in the mouth as often as five times a day.

Spiritus Melissae comp. dilution
For internal use: take 10 drops in water or on a sugar cube in the case of feeling unwell, frightened, over-emotional or weak.
For external use: apply to the forehead in case of headache.

Liquids for external use / ointments

Arnica essence for external use
An important remedy for all types of contusion when there are no open wounds; consult the chapter on trauma for how to use this remedy.

Arnica wet wipes
To use as first aid in the case of contusion, such as bruises and insect bites; apply locally in the form of a pack and hold in place for a long time. Bind even with an ordinary handkerchief.

Arnica planta tota ointment 30%
A remedy that can replace the previous one in the case of trauma, sprains and joint or muscle pain.

Arnica/Urtica dilution for external use
Arnica/Urtica ointment
A fundamental remedy for burns, scalds and insect bites. Consult the relevant chapters for how to use this remedy.

Calendula essence dilution for external use
Calendula/Salbe ointment 10%
The dilution, a teaspoon in a glass of water, is useful for application onto wounds and skin infections since it promotes wound healing. For minor abrasions, nappy rash (if more acute use the essence in the form of a pack) and cutaneous inflammations, apply the ointment twice a day directly onto the skin or on a dry gauze. Use the dilution for mouthwashes and gargles in the case of gingivitis.

Levisticum ear drops
In the case of earache, introduce the oil, warmed to 37°C in a *bain marie*, in-

to the auditory canal from one to three times a day. Otherwise, dip a small rolled up plug of cotton in the warmed oil and introduce it into the auditory canal: repeat several times a day (see the chapter on earache).

Mercurialis comp. ointment
This is useful for all types of wounds, in particular for abscesses and infected wounds that are slow to heal; it can also be used for some forms of dermatitis or eczema. Apply directly or on a gauze onto the injured part two or three times a day.

Arnica oil (Arnika-Massageöl)
Use in the case of muscle pain, colds, limb pain and also to warm muscles before sporting activities.

Plantago comp. ointment
Rub the balsam once or twice day on the chest and back in the case of catarrhal inflammations of the airways and cough; do not apply to the face of small children, particularly around the nose. On rare occasions this remedy may provoke local reactions because it contains camphor and eucalyptus; for this reason it is not advised for use in children under three years old.

Plantago lanceolata ointment 10%
Use for small or delicate children and those with a sensitive skin.

Suppositories to keep in the home

Aconitum/China comp. suppositories (paediatric suppositories)
Use to promote the restoration of an equilibrium between the "I" and the sensory organs during flu-like illnesses accompanied by fever; this remedy protects against the consequences of high fever. An enema should always be given before using these suppositories.

Echinacea/Mercurius comp. suppositories (paediatric suppositories)
Use in the case of localised inflammatory processes accompanied by fever, such as an acute sore throat or abscesses; it is always useful to give an enema first in order to increase the efficacy of the stimulus to the intestinal immune system.

Herbal teas to keep in the home

Chamomile flowers (preparation for tea)
Useful for teas but also for packs in the case of painful abdominal cramps due to gastrointestinal disorders and in the case of cystitis; a warm pack is also useful for windy colic in the neonate. The tea should be drunk directly without adding anything, not even sugar.

Lime blossom (preparation for tea)
Use this marvellous sweat-inducing tea for every type of cold (see the chapters on fever, colds and influenza).

Sage leaves (preparation for tea)
Sage tea (Salvia Officinalis, blue sage) with added fresh lemon juice can be used for gargles in the case of sore throat and gingivitis.

Injectable vials to keep in the home

Arnica planta tota D3 vial
Echinacea/Argentum injectable solution
Silicea comp. injectable solution
These ampoules for injection are only listed to meet the needs of a doctor. Keep a *box of disposable insulin syringes* in the home because the contents of the vials are administered by subcutaneous injection.

Warnings
It is important to store herbs in glass jars. Label the jars, tubes, etc. in order to avoid errors. Store the remedies in a cool, dark place, but only in the refrigerator if specifically instructed.
Oils must be disposed of when they become rancid. Dried herbs last for one solar year at most and must, therefore, be replaced each year. After three years ointments are less effective and should be replaced.

Information on anthroposophic medicine

Useful information on anthroposophic medicine worldwide can be found at the website of the Medical Section of the School of Spiritual Science at the Goetheanum:
www.medsektion-goetheanum.org

The Medical Section is the hub of the whole anthroposophic medical movement. Fundamentally, it provides:
– post-graduate medical specialisation;
– training of paramedical staff;
– coordination of educational and research activities.
The body coordinating the individual medical associations is the International Federation of Anthroposophic Medical Associations (IVAA):
www.ivaa.info

General Anthroposophical Society
For more general information on anthroposophy and on the General Anthroposophical Society, visit or contact:
www.goetheanum.org
sekretariat@goetheanum.org
Address:
General Anthroposophical Society
Rüttiweg 45
CH-4143 Dornach 1
Switzerland
Tel. +41 (0)61 706 42 42
Fax +41 (0)61 706 43 14

Bibliography

Fundamental works by Rudolf Steiner

*The German Edition of Rudolf Steiner's Collected Works — the Gesamtausgabe (GA) published by Rudolf Steiner Verlag, Dornach, Switzerland — includes about 350 titles, organized either by type of work (written or spoken), chronology, audience (public or other), or by subject (education, art, medicine, and so on). For ease of comparison, the Collected Works in English (**CW**) follows the German exactly.*

Steiner Rudolf, *The Philosophy of Freedom. The Basis for a Modern World Conception* (CW 4). Also published as: *Intuitive Thinking as a Spiritual Path*. Philosophical analysis of human freedom and morality.

Steiner Rudolf, *Theosophy. An Introduction to the Supersensible Knowledge of the World and the Destination of Man* (CW 9). An introduction to the spiritual processes in human life and in the cosmos.

Steiner Rudolf, *Knowledge of the Higher Worlds. How is it Achieved?* (CW 10). A modern path of initiation.

Steiner Rudolf, *Occult Science. An Outline* (CW 13). Also published as: *An Outline of Esoteric Science*. Overview of the vast processes of cosmic evolution and humanity's place within them.

Steiner Rudolf, *The Renewal of the Social Organism* (CW 23). Also published as: *Towards Social Renewal. Basic Issues of the Social Question*. Explains the need for fundamental changes to the way we organize society.

Books by Rudolf Steiner about Anthroposophic Medicine

Steiner Rudolf, Wegman Ita, *Fundamentals of Therapy. An Extension of the Art of Healing through Spiritual-Scientific Knowledge* (CW 27), Mercury Press, Spring Valley, NY, 1999. This small book is, as the title rightly says, the fundamental work on anthroposophic medicine, written in collaboration between Rudolf Steiner and Dr. Ita Wegman, a pioneer of anthroposophic medicine.

Steiner Rudolf, *Transforming the Soul* (CW 58/59), vols. 1 & 2, Rudolf Steiner Press, 2006. Also published as: *Metamorphoses of the Soul/Paths of Experience*, vols. 1 & 2, Rudolf Steiner Press, 1983.

Steiner Rudolf, *An Occult Physiology* (CW 128 - Prague, March 20-28, 1911), Rudolf Steiner Press, 2005.

Steiner Rudolf, *Spiritual Science and Medicine* (CW 312), Rudolf Steiner Press., London. Also published as: *Introducing Anthroposophical Medicine.*

Steiner Rudolf, *Anthroposophical Spiritual Science and Medical Therapy* (CW 313 - Dornach, April 11-18, 1921), Mercury Press, 1991.

Steiner Rudolf, *Physiology and Therapy Based on Spiritual Science* (CW 314). Healthcare can only arise from knowledge of the spiritual reality of mankind and is a shared characteristic of doctors, teachers and politicians.

Steiner Rudolf, *Physiology and Therapeutics: Four lectures* (CW 314 - Dornach, October 7-9, 1920), Mercury Press, 1986.

Steiner Rudolf, *The Anthroposophical Approach to Medicine* (CW 314 - Stuttgart, October 26-28, 1922), Anthroposophic Publishing Company, 1951.

Steiner Rudolf, *Eurythmy Therapy* (CW 315 - Dornach, April 12-18, 1921; Stuttgart, October 28, 1922), Rudolf Steiner Press., 2009.

Steiner Rudolf Course for Young Doctors, (*Meditative Contemplations and Instructions for Deepening the Art of Healing*) (CW 316). Includes: the Christmas Course; the Easter Course; and *The Bridge between Universal Spirituality and the Physical Constitution of Man*, Mercury Press, 1994.

Steiner Rudolf, *Education for Special Needs* (CW 317 - Dornach, June 25-July 12, 1924). Rudolf Steiner Press., London,1998. The basis and beginning of anthroposophic special needs education.

Steiner Rudolf, *Broken Vessels: The Spiritual Structure of Human Frailty* (CW 318). Anthroposophic Press, 2003. Also published as: *Pastoral Medicine*, Anthroposophic Press, 1987.

Steiner Rudolf, *The Healing Process: Spirit, Nature & Our Bodies* (CW 319 - Various cities, August 28, 1923-August 29, 1924), Anthroposophic Press, 2000. Presents the fundamental principles of anthroposophic medical practice and remedies to a non-medical public.

Steiner Rudolf, *From Comets to Cocaine: Lectures to the Workmen*, (CW 348 - Dornach, October 19, 1922-February 10, 1923), Rudolf Steiner Press, 2000. Themes of health and illness as presented to the builders working on the Goetheanum.

Works by other authors

Bentheim (van) T., Bos S, Visser W., Houssaye (de la) E., *Caring for the Sick at Home,* SteinerBooks, Inc, 1989. A valuable book written by a group of Dutch anthroposophic nurses and a midwife. It contains some very clear, simple instructions on external anthroposophic treatments and how to care for a sick person at home. It is an ideal, practical companion to this book.

Evans Michael, Rodger Iain, *Anthroposophical Medicine: Healing for Body, Soul and Spirit*, Floris Books, 1998. This book, written by a dear English colleague, is useful for exploring in more depth some concepts of anthroposophic medicine, particularly those concerning the theoretical and practical basis of diagnosis and treatment; a helpful introduction to the works by Steiner.

Mees Eva (*et alii*), *Anthroposophische Kunsttherapie*, Urachhaus, 2003 (German ed.). A brief treatise on anthroposophic artistic therapies.

Wolff Otto, *Heilmittel für typische Krankheiten*, Freies Geistesleben, 2013 (German ed.). Devoted to the "typical" remedies, often cited in this book, prepared according to the original instructions of Rudolf Steiner: these remedies are an essential component of anthroposophic medicine.

Some books on anthroposophic paediatrics

Glöckler Michaela, Göbel Wolfgang, *A Guide to Child Health*, Floris Books, 2007. (German ed.: *Kindersprechstunde. Ein medizinisch-pädagogischer Ratgeber*, Urachhaus, 2013). An excellent manual on anthroposophic paediatrics for doctors and parents, with useful educational advice.

Holtzapfel Walter, *Krankheitsepochen der Kindheit*, Freies Geistesleben, 1960 (German ed.). A very interesting, easy to read book by one of the first anthroposophic doctors on the importance of childhood illnesses in the development of children. Aimed at doctors, teachers and educators.

Linden (zur) Wilhelm, *A Child Is Born: A Natural Guide to Pregnancy, Birth And Early Childhood*, Rudolf Steiner Press, 2004. A manual of advice written by a great anthroposophic paediatrician.

Some important works on education for children with special needs

Henning Hansmann, *Education for Special Needs: Principles and Practice in Camphill Schools*, Floris Books, 1992.

Lievegoed Bernard, *Heilpädagogische Betrachtungen. Hilfen zur Behandlung von Entwicklungsstörungen*, Freies Geistesleben, 1995 (German ed.).

Lievegoed Bernard, *Phases of Childhood: Growing in Body, Soul and Spirit*, Anthroposophic Press, 1997.

Uhlenhoff Wilhelm, *The Children of the Curative Education Course: Case Studies*, Floris Books, 2009. A follow-up of the children and youngsters of Rudolf Steiner's *"Education for Special Needs"*.

Subject index

abdominal pain, 320
acetone, 71
acne, 217-220
aerophagy, 143-146
ageing, 247, 277
AIDS, 216
– and anorexia, 279
alcohol, 308, 312
allergy, 41, 49, 96-106, 224, 225, 234, 264, 292
– prevention, 102
– to food, 102-104, 107
anaemia, 64, 140, 272, 280-287
– diet in, 286
– in adolescents, *see* chlorosis
– in pregnancy, 281, 284
– iron-deficient, 282
anal fissures, 175-179
anaphylactic shock, 231, 232
angina, 314
animal bites, 230-232
anorexia, 279
– nervosa, 285
anxiety, 288-301
appendicitis, acute, 153, 154
appetite, 184
– decrease in, 276
art therapies, 18, 119, 119n
arthritis, 246, 247
asthenia, *see* tiredness
asthma, 90-92, 94, 101, 114-124, 223
– allergic, 99, 120
– in children, 121
atherosclerosis, 102, 273, 306, 312
athlete's foot, 228
atopy, 120, 122n
atrophy, 273
backache, 246, 257-262
– influences of diet, 260
bacterial flora, alteration of, 45
biliary dyskinesia, 150

bites, 230-232
bladder infection, 88
bloating, *see* aerophagy
body warmth, 16, 17, 34-38
boils, 217-220
breastfeeding, 101, 156, 157
breathing, difficulty in, 75
bronchi, hyperreactivity of, 120
bronchitis, 69, 85, 88, 89, 93, 94, 123, 317, 319
– acute, 90, 91, 93
– asthmatic, 123
– spasmodic, 87, 94
– – asthmatic, 123
bronchopneumonia and loss of appetite, 278
bulimia, 285
burns, 235, 236, 319
caffeine, 308
callouses, 215n, 228
cancer, 18, 177
– and childhood illnesses, 264
– of the breast, 308
candidiasis, 226
cardiac arrhythmias, 282
cardiovascular diseases, 50
catarrh, 61, 73, 84, 86, 87, 89, 92, 123
– bronchial, 117
– prevention, 46, 49
cervical whiplash, 254
CFS, *see* chronic fatigue syndrome
change of air, 183-85, 318
chemotherapy, 38
chicken pox, *see* varicella
chilblains, 229
childhood illnesses, 263-271
chlorosis, 284-286
cholera, 159
cholesterol, concentration in the blood, 170, 210
chronic fatigue syndrome, 272n
cirrhosis of the liver, 175n, 281

Subject index

cold, 57-61, 64, 75, 79, 85, 86, 93, 123, 129, 191, 192, 318, 320
– acute, 56
– catarrhal, 59
– related disorders, 57-61
cold sores, *see* Herpes simplex
colibacillosis, 196
colic
– abdominal, 155
– biliary, 148, 149, 151
– intestinal, 318
– renal, 148, 152, 153
collapse, 159
colon, tumour of, 159
conjunctivitis, 125-128
– allergic, 111, 126, 127
– bacterial, 125
– catarrhal, 125, 126
– dry, 127
– in the neonate, 125
– viral, 126
constipation, 63, 117, 153, 155, 169-174
contusions, 237, 240, 319
cough, 73, 76, 77, 84-95, 117, 120, 123, 320
– acute, 85, 91
– and diet in children, 90
– chronic, 85, 91
– dry, 85, 86, 88, 123
– irritant, 89
– spasmodic, 89
– wet, 86, 90
– whooping, *see* pertussis
cracked skin, 242
Crohn's disease, 163
crushed finger, 238
cut teeth, 59n
cuts, wounds from, 241
– of the skin, 242
cystitis, 88n, 189-199
– acute, 191
– interstitial, 196
– recurrent, 194, 195
dacryocystitis, 128
decalcification, 101

dehydration, 159, 168
dental
– abscess, 134
– caries, 133, 255n
– extractions, 241
depression, 274, 288n
dermatitis, 221-229
– atopic, *see* eczema, atopic or constitutional
– from contact, 224
dialysis, 305
diarrhoea, 155, 159-164, 185, 283
– acute, 160
– traveller's, 165-168
diet
– abuse, 69
– alterations, 184
– disorders of, 285
– food poisoning, 165-168
– in childhood, 39-50
– in the anaemic person, 286
– intolerances, 41, 49, 104, 159, 292
– reflections on backache, 260
– reflections on blood pressure, 310
digestion, 49
disc herniation, 259
dizziness, 282, 283
dysentery, 159n
dysmenorrhoea, 200-202, 318
dyspepsia, 117
dyspnoea, 120
earache, 129-132, 319
eczema, 99, 163, 215, 221-229
– atopic or constitutional, 101, 104, 120, 203, 219
– palpebral, 226
ejaculation, painful, 197
encopresis, 174
endodontitis, *see* pulpitis
enuresis, 186-188
epidemics of influenza, 62, 63
epididymitis, 199
epiglottitis, acute, *see* laryngitis, supraglottic
ethmoiditis, 78
eurhythmy, 313

Subject index

eurhythmy therapy, 18, 119, 119n, 255n
– for backache, 260
– postural treatment, 259
exudative diathesis, 102, 108
fainting, 283, 284n, 318
false croup, *see* laryngitis, subglottic
febrile hallucinations, 55
febrile seizures, 55
fever, 34-38, 52-56, 65, 69, 72, 73, 78, 93, 94, 191, 264, 318, 320
– in abdominal pain, 150
flatulence, *see* meteorism
fluid retention, 192
food intolerance, *see* diet
food poisoning, *see* diet
food pyramid, 310
fright, 237
fungi on the skin, *see* mycosis
ganglioneuritis, *see* Herpes zoster
gastroenteritis, 163, 167
– acute, 162
genital herpes, 208, 211
– inflammation of, 242
German measles, *see* rubella
gingivitis, 74, 136, 319, 320
haematoma, 237, 241, 319
– subungeal, 238
haematuria, 193
haemorrhage, 163, 241, 242, 281
– from haemorrhoids, 175, 177
haemorrhoids, 175-179
hair bulb, obstruction of, 219
hay fever, 98, 99, 101, 107-113, 116, 122n
head injury, 239
headache, 54, 58, 78, 79, 138-143
– catamenial, 141
health and the meaning of life, 299
hearing, disorders of, 18
heart, disorders of, 272, 302n, 307, 311, 313
hepatitis, 121
Herpes simplex, 208-212
Herpes virus, 88n
Herpes zoster, 205-207

– ophthalmic, 206
hoarseness, 93
Hodgkin's lymphoma, 216
hypertension, 19, 302-314
– arterial, 119n
– in the menopause, 305
– portal, 175n
hypertrophic scarring, *see* keloid
hypokalaemia, 159
hypotension (low blood pressure), 64, 159, 305, 306
impetigo, 203, 204, 208, 219
infarction, 245n, 305
infections, 45
– intestinal, *see* intestine
– viral, 52
inflammation
– catarrhal, 320
– gastrointestinal, *see* gastroenteritis
– intestinal, *see* intestine
– of the urinary tract, 318
influenza, 59, 62-67, 318, 320
– contagion, 66
– convalescence, 66
– in children, 60
insect stings, 230-232
insomnia, 142, 288-301
intercostal pain, 247
intertrigo, 226
intestine
– air in, *see* meteorism
– blockage, 118
– carcinoma, 177
– cramps, 173
– infections, 159
– inflammation, 154
– stasis, 173
iron
– deficiency of, *see* anaemia
– excess of, 280, 281
irritability, 276
itching of the skin, 221, 222
jet-lag, *see* change of air
joint sprains, 240, 319
joints, pain in, 245-249
keloid, 235, 243

Subject index

kidney, disorder of, 302n
– inflammation, 118
kidney stones, *see* colic, renal
language, disturbance of, 18
laryngitis, 73, 92, 93, 319
– subglottic, 75
– supraglottic, 75
laryngospasm, 76
lethargic encephalitis, 62
liver, 117
lombalgia
– eurhythmy therapy, 260
– psychosomatic, 257n
loss of appetite, 278, 279, 317
– in pregnancy, 279
low back pain, 257-262
lumbago, 257-262
lungs, disorders of, 184
lymphatism, 108
lymphoma, 216
mastoiditis, 129
measles, 121, 122n, 263-266
meningitis, 269
menopause and hypertension, 305
menstruation, 281
– absence of, 27n
– headache and menstrual cycle, 139, 141
– menstrual pain, 200-202, 318
metabolic acidosis, 159
meteorism, 143-146
– in the neonate, 156
migraine, 138, 139, 141, 142
Montezuma's revenge, 165, 165n
movement, disorders of, 245-250
mumps, 122n, 269
muscles
– cramps, 246, 251, 252
– inflammation, 247
– pain, 320
– warm, 320
mycosis, 226-229
myoma in the uterus, 281
myopia, 119n, 255n
nappy rash, 319
nasal secretion, 82, 123

naso-lacrymal duct, obstruction of, 128
nausea, 279, 317
neck pain, 253, 254, 256
neonatal herpes, 208
neuralgia, 192, 247, 262
neurasthenia, 273
neuritis, 192
nickel, eczema due to contact with, 225
nicotine, 307
nutrition, *see* diet
obesity, 307, 308
orchitis, 269
ossification, 105
osteoarthritis, 247-250
otalgia, *see* earache
otitis, 129-132
over-emotional, 319
overnutrition, 42
overwork, 278
Parkinson's disease, 62, 281
parotitis, *see* mumps
pelvic congestion, 176, 177
peritonitis, 154
pertussis (whooping cough), 87, 89, 269-271
pharyngitis, 69, 73, 85, 92, 319
pharyngotracheitis, 73
phlebitis, 180, 181
– of delivery, 182
– post-traumatic, 181
piercing, 225
pneumonia, 15, 16, 58, 92, 93, 95
– atypical (SARS), 184
– viral, 85
posture, prevention with eurhythmy, 259
pregnancy, 102, 268
– and anaemia, 281, 284
– and loss of appetite, 279
protein, excess of, 43-47
psychosomatic and back pain, 257n
pulpitis, 136
pytiriasis versicolor, 226
rheumatism, 245-250

Subject index

rheumatism, influences of diet, 249
rhinitis, 73, 78, 120
– acute, 60
– chronic, 61
rhythmical massage, 119, 119n
ringworm, 226
rubella (German measles), 122n, 268
SARS, see pneumonia, atypical
scalds, 319
scar formation, 241-244, 319
– influence of diet, 243
scarlet fever, 263, 266
sciatica, 259, 262
sclerosis, 39, 45, 46, 50, 247, 277
scoliosis, 18, 19n, 255n
sebaceous glands, infection of, 219
shock, post-traumatic, 237
sinusitis, 54, 58, 61, 77-83, 89, 192
– ethmoidal, 78
– frontal, 78
– maxillary, 78
– prevention, 83
– sphenoidal, 78
skin
– abscess, 135, 219
– disorders, 118, 221
– superficial infections, see impetigo
– tumours, 233
sleep disorders, 288-301
smoking, 307
sore throat, see throat, sore
Spanish 'flu, epidemic, 62, 63
spasm, 115
– abdominal, 318
– anal, 178
spleen, 118
splenectomy, 118
St. Anthony's fire, see Herpes zoster
stings, 230-232
stomach
– air in, see aerophagy
– ache, 147-158
stomatitis, 192, 226, 318
stones
– in the gallbladder, 149
– in the ureter, 152

stress, 115, 279, 282
stroke, 240, 302n, 308
sty, 128
sun, exposure to, 233, 234
sunburn, 233, 234
surgery, 237-244
tachycardia, 124
teeth
– dentition, 134
– disorders, 133-137
– extraction, 136
– hygiene, 133
– neuralgic tooth pain, 133
tendinitis, 130
tenesmus of the bladder, 192, 193
testicle, inflammation of, see orchitis
tetany, 159
thinness, pathological, 184
throat angina, in children, 147, 147n
throat, sore, 68-74, 92, 93, 147n, 318
– in children, 71
thrush (mycosis), 226
thyroid disorder, 282
tinea versicolor, 226
tiredness, 272-279
– and art therapy, 273, 274
– in the elderly, 277
tonsillectomy, 155
tonsillitis, 69, 71, 72, 74, 129, 317, 319
toothache, see teeth
torticollis, 253-256
tracheitis, 69, 85, 89, 92, 93, 95
tracheobronchitis, 91, 92
trauma, 237-244
– emotional, 318
– physical, 318
tuberculosis, 184
– primary, 121
tumour, 38, 50, 79, 83, 102, 159, 233, 272, 281
tympanum, rupture of, 131
typhus, 159
ulcer, 148
– of the duodenum, 163
– of the stomach, 163
ulcerative colitis, 32, 163

Subject index

undernutrition, 42
urethritis, 198
urethrocystitis, 198
urinary bladder, inflammation of, *see* cystitis
urination
– burning, 191-193, 242
– frequency, 197
– pain, 197
– stimulus, 191, 197
urine, blood in, *see* haematuria
urticaria, 99, 120
uterine cervix, infection of, 199
vaccination, 122n, 216, 264

vaginal fornix, infection of, 199
varicella (chicken pox), 205, 267, 269
varicose veins, 180-182
verruca, 213-216
visual disorders, 18
vomiting, 148, 158, 159, 163, 167, 168
weakness, 276
weight loss, 276
whitlow, 219
whooping cough, *see* pertussis
windy colic in the neonate, 156, 157, 318
wounds, 241-244, 319, 320
– bleeding, 240

A NOTE FROM RUDOLF STEINER PRESS

We are an independent publisher and registered charity (non-profit organisation) dedicated to making available the work of Rudolf Steiner in English translation. We care a great deal about the content of our books and have hundreds of titles available – as printed books, ebooks and in audio formats.

As a publisher devoted to anthroposophy...

- We continually commission translations of previously unpublished works by Rudolf Steiner and invest in re-translating, editing and improving our editions.

- We are committed to making anthroposophy available to all by publishing introductory books as well as contemporary research.

- Our new print editions and ebooks are carefully checked and proofread for accuracy, and converted into all formats for all platforms.

- Our translations are officially authorised by Rudolf Steiner's estate in Dornach, Switzerland, to whom we pay royalties on sales, thus assisting their critical work.

So, look out for Rudolf Steiner Press as a mark of quality and support us today by buying our books, or contact us should you wish to sponsor specific titles or to support the charity with a gift or legacy.

office@rudolfsteinerpress.com
Join our e-mailing list at www.rudolfsteinerpress.com

RUDOLF STEINER PRESS